God's Original Diet

The Spiritual Way to Health

God's Original Diet

The Spiritual Way to Health

Dr. Malcolm Hill

Wright Book
Fayetteville, Georgia

Wright Books®
A Division of
Wright Publishing
Atlanta, GA

Information address:

Wright Publishing, Inc.
320 DeVilla Trace
Fayetteville, GA 30214

Library of Congress Control Number
2006900955

Dr. Malcolm Hill

First Edition

Printed in the U.S.A.   ISBN 0-935087-29-X

Cover Design by Cleveland Clements

Author's Note

The opinions you are about to read are those of Dr. Malcolm Hill. When seeking health advice, always consult a healthcare physician. In the event you use information in this book without your doctor's approval, you are prescribing for yourself, which is your constitutional right, but the publisher and the author assume no responsibility. Remember it is not God's will for you to be sick.

Heavenly Father, We thank you for your faithfulness. We know that our Lord is a faithful God who keepeth covenant and mercy with them that love him and keep his commandments to a thousand generations. Lord if we are faithless yet you remain faithful; you cannot deny your word. You promised in your word that while the earth remaineth, seed time and harvest, and cold and heat, and summer and winter, and day and night shall not cease. You created the four seasons for a reason, but Oh God, we thank you for spring time; and a time for new beginnings and new growth and most of all new life. We pray for Dr. Malcolm Hill as he receives revelation concerning health. Holy Father, I ask that you may bless each reader of this book as they step into a new life of better health for themselves and their families. We ask these blessings in Jesus name. Amen.

Prayer by Patricia Hill

This book is dedicated to all of God's children who are tired of being defeated in the area of their health. From this day forth there will be no more sickness in your body. The generational curse of sickness in your family stops today.

Acknowledgments

I would like to thank God for giving me this ministry. I feel honored to be chosen to teach the ministry of health.

I would like to thank my Dad and Mom, Haile and Patricia, for their love, support, and discipline. When I was a lad I thought you were strict but now I realize you were the best parents a child can have. Love you.

To my brothers, Terrance and Corey, thanks for your love, support, and that big-brotherly advice.

To my best friend, Dr. Royce McGowan, thanks for your support and encouragement.

Special thanks to everyone who has been a positive inspiration in my life - school teachers, college professors, natural hygienic physicians, friends, and family, etc.

Thanks to Dr. Jay DiVagno who has truly been God sent in my life. Thanks for being my mentor.

Thanks to Pastor Chris Bowen and Living Faith Tabernacle Church. You have been supportive and open to this ministry when others were not.

Finally, another special thanks goes to my Mom. I would like to thank you for your fasting and prayer. I realize it is your fasting and prayer that keeps our family blessed and for that I want to say thanks.

The doctor of the future will give no medicine but will interest his patients in the care of the human frame, in diet, and in the cause and prevention of disease.

– Thomas A. Edison

I met Dr. Hill several years ago. He's a warm and caring man with a passion for knowledge and information to help people make choices that will give them back their health and a better quality of life.

I've personally experienced and seen many people have amazing results through the water fast under Doctor supervision.

Read this book and then come to your own conclusions. You'll never feel the same about the food you eat.

– Linda Evans
Actor on Dynasty and Big Valley

FOREWORD

As Senior Pastor of Living Faith Tabernacle for the past 16 years, I have had many church members tell me that my sermons have "stepped all over their toes." Although it is true that sometimes, the truth hurts, as Christians, we also realize that it is the TRUTH that sets us free! (John 8:32).

In his book, ***God's Original Diet, The Spiritual Way to Health,*** Dr. Malcolm Hill touches on some areas that are very sensitive, especially for the Body of Christ. We are so used to having our homecoming dinners, fellowship meetings, and celebrations that are centered around food, and we don't want anyone coming in our churches telling us that some of the foods we consider to be "staples" of the human diet can actually be harming us, or even possibly shortening our lives.

Just as God had a Divine plan for the world when He designed it, He also had plan for us to live healthy, vibrant lives. If we would stick to His plan, we would find ourselves without so many health and dietary issues today, such as high cholesterol, high blood pressure, obesity, sugar diabetes, etc. that are sometimes simply brought on by our own habits and lifestyles.'

Please open your heart and mind to receive the revelation God has given Dr. Hill through this book. I have personally experienced and have heard testimonies of others who have put his teachings into practice and were able to naturally reverse health problems they had struggled with for years, simply by putting the right foods in their bodies.

It is Dr. Hill's passion to see God's people thrive and prosper with good health and long life. Make these principles become alive in your heart and you will see how God can transform you both physically and spiritually through this powerful ministry.

Chris Bowen, Sr. Pastor
Living Faith Tabernacle
Forest Park, GA

TABLE OF CONTENTS

Introduction

There have been many people who have prevented and reversed sickness in their body by changing their diet to eating a majority of God's Original Diet. This diet along with living a healthy spiritual lifestyle is usually enough to prevent many diseases that man is afflicted with today.

Using Biblical principal's everyday in the area of health is the safest and most effective way to prevent and reverse diseases. I have seen many suffering with diabetes, high blood pressure, obesity, uterine fibroids, arthritis and even early stages of cancer reverse these illnesses by eating the way God intended.

You too after reading this book can learn to live an abundant life without sickness just as God intended for you. I do not worry about sickness anymore because I have decided to eat the way God instructed me and God wants the same for you. It is not God's will for you to be suffering within a sick body; it is not God's will for you to be taking unnecessary drugs and it is not God's will for you to die before your time.

But first we have to adress why sickness occurs and then change the cause of sickness instead of covering up the symptoms with medicine. Only when you change to living a lifestyle supported by God will you come into abundant life. This book will show you the way. Congratulations on making the steps toward Spiritual Health.

The Foundation for Dr. Hill's Teachings

God's Original Diet   -vs-   **Man-Made Foods**

Healthy Foods are:
1. Fruits
2. Vegetables
3. Raw Nuts and Seeds
4. Whole Grains
5. Legumes
6. Water

These are all earth-grown
Living foods and they
are provided by God

Unhealthy Foods are:
1. Fast Foods
2. Refined Processed Foods
3. Salt, Sugar, Dairy
4. Excessive Meats
5. Alcohol and Tobacco
6. Coffee, Sodas, Tea, Kool-Aid

These are all
Dead foods and they are
provided by man

If a majority of your diet consists of healthy foods then you will be blessed with health, but if a majority of your diet consists of unhealthy foods then you may be cursed with sickness and die before your time.

I.
Why God's Children Get Sick

The Country Life

Growing up in a small country town in Mississippi, there was little to do, and getting into trouble was hard. Going to school was the most exciting thing to do. I hated when the school year was over, because there wasn't much to do at home but work.

My family was a little different from other families in that my mother was very strict. It seemed as though our neighbors and friends experienced many things that my brothers and I could not. There were some places we could not go, some things on television we could not watch, and some things we could not say in front of our parents. For fun, I would ride my bike, fish, or play basketball. I could not wait to grow up and become a man. I was tired of the boring country life and could not wait to get away.

My parents were, and still are, also deeply spiritual in that they walk very close to God. My brothers and I went to church *every* Sunday until we were old enough to go off to college.

My mother provided the love and the rules of the house. She disciplined my brothers and me with what she called the 'razor strap'. It was made of three extension cords braided like a little girl's hair. The razor strap was the best way to keep my brothers and I out of trouble.

My father worked hard and provided food and shelter for the family. He barely had a high school education, but he was a very hard worker and taught us the rules of life. He taught us the difference between good and bad, that nothing in life is easy, and that you have to work hard for what you get. He also believed in growing his own food. Every year he would plant a big garden, and at the end of the garden season the family had enough food to last us until the next garden season.

My brothers and I would always get mad when the garden season came around, because we knew we had to work. I can recall working in the garden as my friends were riding their bikes and playing. I would just look at them and wish I could play with them, but I had work to do. They would sometimes tease me because I was always working and not playing with them.

Sometimes, when we had to go and hoe the fields of peas, butterbeans, and other vegetables, we would chop some of them down and bury them in the dirt just so we wouldn't have to hoe them the next week. I can remember my dad telling mom that the garden was looking thinner than the week before. He just believed deer, rabbits, coyotes, or other animals were eating the plants. If he had known we chopped and buried the vegetables, we would have gotten the razor strap.

When the peas and butterbeans were ready to be harvested, my dad would pick them. My mom, brothers, and I would shell the peas and butterbeans all day. Sometimes we shelled peas and butterbeans for so long that our fingers and thumbs turned purple. This made us mad. We could not wait to leave home. Little did we know, those were the best days of our lives.

We ate more than the food our father grew in the garden. We also bought food from grocery stores - meats and some fruits and vegetables that our soil could not grow. However, the majority of the food we ate did come from our garden. As I grew up, I realized how healthy my family was compared to other families in the community and elsewhere. It was common for people in my community to suffer strokes or heart attacks, to be diabetic, and have high blood pressure. Why was that? My mom explained that it was because our family was close to the Lord, and that He shunned sickness and disease away from our family. However, I knew many other people that served the Lord and still had heart disease, cancer, diabetes, and other diseases.

Growing up, my mom always told me to ask God for wisdom, and I did. I found out that wisdom is usually just common sense.

During my college years I had to come home for a funeral of a family member almost twice a year. These people were not my immediate family, and they were dying off fast. The family had no clue what was happening. Other family members and I began to become fearful. "God, what is going on? Almost all of my aunts and uncles are dying of cancer. Is the family cursed? Is the family carrying a cancer gene? Is this what I have to look forward to? Teach me what is going on," I asked God.

"God, Why Do We Get Sick?"

I enrolled in Chiropractic School because the teachings were similar to those I grew up with. My mother did not believe in putting an aspirin in my mouth just because I had a headache. She did not give me cough syrup just because I had a cold or seek surgery because my tonsils were inflamed. At this particular school the Lord led me to the teaching of a man who was a Natural Hygienist. He taught me that health comes from the inside out, not outside in. He taught me that everyone is in charge of his or her own health.

We make ourselves sick. There is no gene that gives you obesity, cancer, heart disease, or any other disease. You don't automatically get diseases because you're old, and sickness is not something you have to live with. Just because a father or mother had a disease does not mean that their children will develop it. Yes, if you live the same lifestyle and eat the same foods as they did, you will have the same sickness as your parents. I learned that the foods you eat play the most important role in determining your health. A healthy diet is a diet that causes no disease. I find that people think they are eating a healthy diet because their doctor told them they were, or they saw a particular food on television advertised as healthy.

My opinion of health is totally different than other doctors' opinions. A healthy body is a body free of disease and in good shape. A healthy body does not need drugs in order to function. A healthy body does not need vitamins in the form of a pill to live. Americans have been brainwashed to believe that eating dead foods is healthy eating. Nutritionists should be taught to teach the value of foods. Nutritionists should teach that foods that provide the best and most fuel to the body are the healthiest foods, and the foods with the greatest value to humans are the foods that grow from the earth.

So my mom was partially right when she said our family was not sick because our family was close to God. The other reason is because we ate a majority of the foods that God intended for man to eat. I grew up in a community where everyone raised their own food and animals. People in my community raised mostly pigs, cows, and chickens. They were raised and then killed to have meat for the winter.

My community also loved the taste of deer. Every time deer season came around someone would get shot or killed in a deer hunting accident. Many times the deer was not eaten; it was killed for the excitement of the hunt or for the trophy. After killing animals, we would preserve their muscles, what humans call meat, with salt, sulfur, and other harmful chemicals. We would season our vegetables with these meats, especially the pig, in the form of bacon, fatback, ham hock, or pig's feet.

Everyone in my community grew up on the pig. When a pig was killed in the neighborhood the whole community would come around and feast. Every part of the pig would be eaten. Nothing went to waste. We would eat organs that most people would not think of eating - the pig's brain, feet, tail, ears, and head. We would even eat the pig's intestines and its testicles, which we called chitlins and mountain oysters. We would even make a fire, cut the pig's skin, and boil it in fatty grease. We called the pig skin "crackling". The only thing that was not used for food was the blood of the pig. We ate pig, cow, or chicken at every meal - sausage and bacon for breakfast, hamburger for lunch, and chicken for dinner.

When I would eat dinner with the different people in the neighborhood, the meals would be mostly meats and hardly any vegetables and the vegetables that were eaten were seasoned with meats. We would drink tea, coffee, Kool-aid or sodas; never water. There were barbecues almost every weekend. Any occasion was a good reason to barbecue. Many people were suffering from obesity, high blood pressure, cancers, diabetes, strokes, and other illnesses, but at the time, I was too young to understand why. I did not understand anything about the illnesses either.

When someone died in the community, they always died with a disease; they never lived out a normal lifespan. Cancer, diabetes, and heart disease were the top three killers in my community, just as they are in the United States. It seemed like every month someone I knew dropped dead of a heart attack or stroke. Sometimes these were young people. I didn't understand that the food choices we were making were killing us. Now that I have grown up, I understand that the food choices a person makes early in life effects his or her health later in life. Most people are not aware of this until it is too late. We eat, drink, and are merry until the doctor says that we have cancer, or that we have to go on dialysis. When we hear this we try to make a change, but sometimes it is too late.

Follow My Word

I was inspired to write this book because I feel God is tired of seeing His children live their lives in sickness. God is tired of seeing his children die before their time. I have heard many people say that when it's your time to die, that it's just your time. They put the situation on the Lord, saying when the Lord wants you He will take you. This is true to a certain extent, but many people die before their time and speed up the process of dying with unhealthy living and eating. Most people are not aware of the deadly life choices they make. Most of us simply don't know that the foods we eat will either give us life, or take life away from us.

I wrote this book because God wants to clear things up for His children, they are dying and they don't know why. God is tired of His people dying. Millions of people get in the prayer line at church on Sunday. They are sick and want prayer for their illness.

Reading this book will help you know what foods are healthy and which are not.

I want to teach you how to stay out of the doctor's office unless you are in an emergency life-threatening situation. You will learn that it is not God's will for you to be sick, nor is it the devil's fault. It may be due to your food choices and your lifestyle. I don't care about what you have been brainwashed in the past to believe. I don't care if you are Jew or Gentile. I don't care if you are black, white, Asian, Hispanic, or any other ethnic background. I don't care what your blood type is. I don't even care what your religion is. If you eat the way God intended, you will be blessed with good health.

This book will teach you why grandmother died of a stroke, why grandpa died of a heart attack, and why aunt has diabetes. I will tell you why men are dropping dead of heart attacks while they are young. I will teach you how man gets common diseases and how we can prevent them.

It is not God's will for his children to be sick. Earlier, I wrote that I knew many people who were Christians and served God with all their heart, but they were still sick. Think about that statement. There is something wrong with that picture. Why are we children of God, and sick? Sickness is not of God. I know preachers who have different types of cancer, heart disease, or obesity and they serve God with all their hearts. This is another question that I asked God. Lord why is this? He let me know that there are some things we have to do on our own. This means that we are in charge of our own health. Just like we are responsible for living right in order to go to heaven, we are responsible for our health, our food choices and lifestyles. God gave us instructions on how to eat in the beginning of time when he spoke to Adam in Genesis 1:29. It is up to us to live by this law. **"And God said, Behold I have given you every herb bearing seed, which is upon the face of all the earth, and every tree, in the which, is the fruit of the tree yielding seed; to you it shall be for meat."** This law still stands today and will forever stand. We suffer from diseases today because we neglect to follow the law. This law is very easy to understand. We should be eating a majority of foods that grow from the earth.

These are the only life-giving foods, and God made them for his children to eat. The only healthy foods that we eat today are the foods that God intended for us to eat. These foods are fruits, vegetables, raw nuts and seeds, fresh legumes, and whole grains. If God did not make it grow from the earth, it should not be eaten in excessive amounts. We were made from the earth, so it makes sense to eat foods that grow from the earth.

Now I know that some Bible scholars reading this will ask about the book of Leviticus - when God gave Moses and the children of Israel permission to eat certain animals. What about when Jesus fed fish to people in the New Testament? I am not asking you to become a vegetarian. But I am saying that the majority of your diet, ninety percent, should consist of fruits, vegetables, and other earth-grown foods. I feel that you should not eat animals in excess, and some animals should not be eaten at all. God gives us permission to eat animals, but we are eating them, along with other unhealthy foods, in excess. For this we are paying a price with sickness and disease.

God is tired of his people being confused about health. Every month a new vitamin pill is on the market, claiming that it can do wonders. Every year a new diet is advertised, claiming it will help you loose weight. Every week there is a new man-made diet pill, claiming it will help you lose weight. God is tired of his children falling for these lies. I write to you not trying to sell you anything, but to promote the one and only true diet. This diet has been around since the beginning of time, and will be here until the end. It was the first diet known to man and will continue to be the only true healthy diet known to man. It is called, God's Original Diet. Eating this diet will give you all the vitamins, minerals, herbs, and medicine that the body needs. If you are looking for health, then God's Original Diet is the right diet for you. Health comes from healthy living, healthy eating, and a healthy lifestyle. This means your doctor, pastor, family - no one can give you good health. Ultimately, everyone is in charge of his or her own health. You are your own doctor.

Luke 4:23 And God said unto them, Physician heal thyself.

II.
MY PEOPLE ARE DESTROYED
FOR LACK OF KNOWLEDGE

From Birth To A Life of Disease

Let's start with the birth of the average baby. They are usually born in a hospital atmosphere where the doctors and nurses are trying to speed the birth process up as fast as they can, so they can go play golf. The baby is delivered with drugs, naturally, or by c-section, and don't forget about the pulling and twisting of the baby's head during the delivery. As soon as the baby is born, instead of letting nature take its course, man starts to rush things. The baby should have adequate time to let blood flow from the umbilical cord into its body, and after that, the baby will start to breathe naturally on its own. Instead, after the birth, the umbilical cord is cut, and the baby is smacked on the buttocks and has to gasp for air in order to breathe.[1] We all know that when we become frightened we start to breathe fast and take light breaths. This process is not normal. A baby does not breathe normally when it is smacked on the buttocks.

This is a traumatic experience for the baby. It becomes frightened and gasps for air. The breaths the baby takes from then on are fast and light. This is not the way we should breathe. In a normal situation, after the blood flows from the mother's umbilical cord to child, the baby naturally starts to breathe on its own. It does not need a slap on the buttocks in order to breathe. Babies that are allowed to breathe on their own, breathe slow and deep. This is the way we should normally breathe. Humans are naturally, slow and deep breathers. We should breathe slow and deep from the belly, not fast and light from the chest. If you were smacked on the buttocks at birth to make you breathe, you are probably breathing from your chest.

Start taking slow and deep breaths and feel how good and relaxed you become. We are the only animals that have to smack our babies in order to get them to breathe. Cows, lions, and other animals don't have to hit their babies in order to make them breathe. They start to breathe on their own naturally. What makes us different? All animals that are fast breathers have a short lifespan, whereas animals that breathe slowly and deeply have long life spans. Try taking deep breaths in the mornings when you awake and before bedtime, and feel your body relax.

After coming into the world breathing incorrectly, due to a traumatic experience of birth, we get our first meal. Many mothers don't breast-feed, so the baby's first meal is dried up cow's milk in the form of formula. Some are fed plain cow's milk. Cow's milk has no business being fed to adults, not to mention infants. Cow's milk does not benefit humans. I know we are brainwashed to believe that it is one of nature's finest foods; it is, if you are a calf. We are told it is a good source of calcium to help build a baby's bones, and it is, if the baby is a calf. God made cow's milk for calves, dog's milk for puppies, cat's milk for kittens, and human milk for infants. There is a reason a mother starts to produce milk when she is pregnant - it is to feed her newborn. You will never see a cat drinking dog's milk, a lion drinking tiger's milk, or a cow drinking human's milk. These animals are in touch with nature and drink only the milk that nature provides for them to drink.

Milk serves two purposes. It serves as the only source of food that should be given to newborns and babies, and most importantly, it provides a way to pass vitamins, minerals, proteins, hormones, antibodies, and other important nutrients from the mother to the baby.[2,3] This helps to develop a strong immune system in newborns. All the antibodies that the mother has made through the years from fighting off colds and flu and other illness are passed to the baby so that the baby can defend itself from the illnesses its mother had.

If you have a child who constantly catches colds, has problems with ear infections, allergies and asthma and is sickly, it may be because the child was not breast-fed.[4,5] A child that is not breast-fed is far more likely to get an illness than a child who has been breast-fed. Breast-fed babies are healthier because they have antibodies, passed to them from their mothers, to help fight off viruses and bacteria. Babies that are fed cow's milk have the vitamins, minerals, antibodies, and other nutrients passed to them that calves need to be healthy. When we feed our babies cow's milk, they are getting all the nutrients cows need to fight off diseases that cow's have. May I ask, does your baby look like a calf?

If it does not look like a calf, give your baby mother's milk to drink. If a mother does not breast-feed her baby it may cause problems for the baby in the future. Women have many excuses for not breast-feeding, including, "it hurts," or "I don't have enough time," or "I'm embarrassed." We should want to give our babies the best, and mother's milk is the best.

After our children get a little older, they start to move on to solid foods. You may buy your toddler different baby food that has been watered down with harmful chemicals. Toddlers are starting to grow teeth at this point, and their teeth and jaw muscles need to be exercised. They cannot learn to chew with and exercise their jaw muscles with liquid food. The baby food you buy from stores can be made in your home from natural foods. You can put the fruit or vegetables in a blender yourself without all the harmful chemicals added. Allow your baby to bite on small pieces of fruit so they can exercise and develop their chewing muscles.

After eating baby food for awhile, our babies can eat cereal. We give them sugar-coated cereals that have no nutritional value. They are processed with very harmful chemicals and sugar. We top it off by pouring cow's milk into it. Cereal companies target our children. They know kids have to get hooked on sweets while they are young if they are going to be hooked on sugar for life. I know cereal is another food we have been brainwashed to believe is good for us, but it is not. When we eat cereal we confuse our body. We are eating a solid food with a liquid. When we eat and drink at the same time, our gastrointestinal tract cannot break down the food properly because the liquid waters it down. Our body starts to produce an enzyme to break down the cereal, but the milk we add to the cereal mixes with the enzyme and dilutes it. When this happens, the sugar-coated cereal is never digested properly. It just sits in the stomach and starts to ferment or form alcohol. This is why some people feel bloated and pass gas after eating cereal with milk.[6] The healthiest cereals are hot cereals such as oatmeal, whole grain grits, millet, and brown rice. Giving your children sugar-coated cereals with cow's milk may be a pre-stage for them to develop diabetes, attention deficit disorder, and many other diseases.[7,8]

After the cereal stage, we start to eat proteins. Of course, we are told that eggs and meat are the best source of protein. We are told meat makes us big and strong. After all, we cannot turn on television without seeing a fast-food commercial trying to influence children to buy their latest special. There is a cute little dog with an accent; there are muppets dressed up as hamburgers, fries, and Coke; there is a cute little girl with different voices advertising a soft drink, all influencing children to buy a product.

As we continue to get older and eat junk foods, our diets start to catch up with us. Most diseases occur around 40 to 50 years of age. This is why most doctors say disease comes with age. I have heard of elderly people going in for a check up and being told by a doctor that they have cancer, sugar diabetes, or heart disease and that it was about time for them to have gotten these diseases because people their age usually do, as if these diseases are a normal part of getting old. Older people tell me all the time not to get old, as if to say, life should stop after 40 years of age. I hear people say that they have arthritis, cancer, and other diseases because they are old. This is the way we are taught to think, but this is far from the truth.

Disease does not come with age. Age should come with wisdom and knowledge.

Just because a lot of people die of heart disease, cancer, strokes, and diabetes does not mean it is normal. It is common, not normal. There are many older people that are in great health. They must have done something right. Our lifestyle while we are young determines our health when we are older.

A Legal Drug Is Still A Drug

> *Ezekiel 47:12 And the fruit shall be for meat (food) and the leaf thereof for medicine.*

Most of man's diseases can be linked to poor diet and living an unhealthy lifestyle. When these diseases occur, we are then encouraged to take medicine. There are some diseases that require medicine, but the majority of diseases don't. We are living in a society that encourages us to take medicine and to never think about what causes sickness in the first place. Commercials come on every minute telling of a pill that will help with a certain condition. When we get a headache, we are taught to take Advil, aspirin, or Tylenol. When we get indigestion, we are taught to take Tums and Pepcid AC. When we are obese, we are taught to go on different diets and take diet pills, which can cost us our lives. It amazes me how we can put someone in jail for selling or using illegal drugs, but we have legal drug stores on almost every corner in America.

Our children can get very confused while watching television. They see one commercial telling them to say no to drugs, and then the next commercial telling them to take Children's Tylenol when they get sick. Parents tell their children to stay away from illegal drugs, while the parent has a multitude of legal drugs in the house. This can confuse children. What is the difference between legal and illegal drugs? They both give you a certain feeling that you desire. They both cover up symptoms. If you want to feel high you smoke, inject, or sniff an illegal drug. If you want to feel sleepy, stimulated, energized, or even get high, you can take a legal drug. There are some legal and illegal drugs that have the same effects on the body.

Marijuana stimulates the central nervous system and speeds up the heart rate; so does caffeine, which is found in coffee, chocolate, teas, and sodas.[9,10] Crack and cocaine cause headaches, anxiety, brain damage, and make you delirious. So does MSG, Monosodium glutamate, found in many canned, Chinese, and seasoned dishes.[11,12] Steroids will cause heart and liver damage and so will aspirin and Tylenol when used in excess.[13,14] Ritalin and Dexedrine given to children with attention deficit disorders cause seizures, anxiety, agitation, and coma, and so do the illegal drugs speed, Ecstasy, and LSD. In fact, Ritalin and Dexedrine are in the same class as speed, Ecstasy, and LSD, meaning they are made of the same ingredients.[15] They all have the same effects. If your kids are taking Ritalin and Dexedrine, they will get the same effects from taking speed, Ecstasy, and LSD.

There are plenty of legal drugs that have the same ingredients as illegal drugs. Who decides which drug is legal or illegal is all part of the political game. There is little difference between legal and illegal drugs. They both have side effects, they both are sold for profit, and they both can have deadly consequences. In fact, legal drugs kill more people than illegal drugs combined, in any given year. Deaths attributed to consumption of tobacco are estimated to be over 400,000 a year, while alcohol adds an additional 200,000 annual deaths. In 2000 there were a reported 17,000 deaths from illegal drugs. This means that over 90% of deaths from substance abuse are attributed to tobacco and alcohol, legal drugs.[16]

If there really is a war on drugs in America, we should eliminate the production of alcohol and tobacco because they kill hundred of thousand times more people than illegal drugs. Aspirin, Tylenol, Ibuprofen, Aleve, and other nonsteroidal anti-inflammatory drugs (NSAIDs) result in approximately 20,000 deaths annually, making it the 15th most common cause of death in the U.S.[17] Whether the drug is legal or illegal, it is still a drug, and can be addictive, so you have to keep coming back for more. I think there is little difference between illegal drug dealers and legal drug dealers. In the world of illegal drugs we have the people who bring the drugs into the country. These are the drug lords who make the most money, and give the drugs to the drug dealers who in turn sell the drugs on the street to the drug users. The drug dealer makes money, and the drug lords make the most money. In the world of legal drugs we have the drug makers, the pharmaceutical companies, who give the drugs to the sellers, doctors. In turn they sell the drugs to the drugs users - you, the public.

Illegal drug dealers have drug houses on street corners where they sell illegal drugs. There is a CVS, Eckerd, and Walgreen's on almost every corner in America where you can buy your legal drugs. When you use an illegal drug for the first time it is usually free, and many samples of drugs from doctors are free also. The doctors make good money and the pharmaceutical companies make great money. There is no difference, except the illegal drug dealer will go to jail if he gets caught. A person addicted to crack has to keep coming back to the drug dealer for more crack to continue to get the feeling they desire. A person also has to go to the doctor's office to get a refill of the particular pill that he or she likes in order to get the feelings they desire.

The top drug dealers are similar to the pharmaceutical companies, illegal drug sellers are similar to doctors and we, the public, are the drug users - whether legal or illegal. We pay our money for their drugs and make the drug sellers and drug manufacturers rich. We are not much different from illegal drug users. They have us hooked like a fish to a pole, just like the crack addict. I know that many people reading this will feel offended, but you must admit, it is the truth.

Costing the average American hundreds of dollars a month, these drug habits are not cheap either. It is sad to have to decide between groceries and legal drugs when all you have to do is eat healthy and exercise. The illegal and legal processes of drug use are the same and most of the time these drugs are not helping the body, only covering up symptoms.

Medicine never eliminates the primary cause of illness. If you have a hole in the roof of your house, and it rains, it will surely rain inside the house. To fix the problem you would not mop up the floor every time it rains. That's like taking an aspirin every time you get a headache. To fix the problem you would repair the roof of the house, that way, it will not rain inside the house again. The hole in the roof is the primary cause. If you were driving your car down a highway and your fuel light came on, you would not spray black paint over the fuel light and just keep riding like everything is ok. That would be covering up the symptom. You would stop the car and put more gas in it. If you drive without filling the car up with gas, it will run out of gas, but if you stop the car and fill it up, the fuel light will go off. Filling the car with gas will eliminate the primary cause. So, if you have a headache every time you don't get enough sleep, would you take an aspirin or get more sleep? If you take the aspirin you are only covering up the symptom of the headache, and you will continue to get headaches. If you get more sleep you have gotten to the primary cause, and you will no longer suffer from headaches.

Just because you have a headache does not mean you need to take an aspirin. Ask yourself what caused the headache? It could be stress, lack of sleep, eating processed sugar (such as candy and soda and other sweets), or coming home to a terrible spouse. Ask yourself what is causing your high blood pressure? It could be from eating excessive amounts of pig, cow, or salt, or a lack of exercise and/or stress. There are many illnesses that could be eliminated if man would remove the primary cause and stop covering up the symptoms of the illness with medicine. You may say, "What is wrong with covering up the symptoms?" All medicine has side effects. Have you noticed that there is always some miracle pill coming on the market every year? I know drugs that are good for arthritis, but they will destroy your liver. There are drugs good for ulcers, but they cause kidney damage. There are drugs used for heart disease, but cause heart palpitations, headaches, and hallucinations. These are not good tradeoffs. When there is a drug used for a certain illness, there will always be side effects. Most drugs have so many side effects that they defeat the purpose of taking them in the first place. The risks of taking them outweigh the benefits. When we cover up symptoms, we are leaving the primary cause active. This could cause serious problems to our health later.

God invented the greatest drug store - the human body. If we live a healthy lifestyle and provide our bodies with healthy foods, it will produce the best medicine. When you cut your finger, your body heals it. Our body fights off germs when we catch a cold or flu. When bacteria invade your body, your body raises its temperature (fever) to kill the bacteria. When we break bones in our body, our bones grow back stronger than before. Our body turns food into energy for survival. The body is the greatest drugstore; we just have to provide it with a good supply of healthy foods and a healthy environment.

Medicine kills many everyday. In fact, the Institute of Medicine (IOM) estimates that medical errors, including adverse reactions to medicines, are the eight leading cause of death among Americans.[18] It does not make sense to me to put my faith in the eighth leading cause of death. There has to be another way, and that way is in the food that we eat. Medicine is in the food that we eat. Foods that grow from the earth have all the medicine our bodies need. If we need certain vitamins, minerals, phytochemicals, or fiber, we can always get them from foods that grow from the earth. These are Mother Nature's and God's medicines, given by God to man to eat. If we eat plenty of these foods, we do not need man's medicine. People who eat excessive amounts of man-made dead foods are the ones who take medicine.

So where does the best source of medicine come from? The earth. We are made from the earth, so the earth has the best source of medicine for us. The best medicine is live vitamins, minerals, phytochemicals, and other nutrients that are found in the earth. The best way to get vitamin A, B, C, and E or any other nutrient, is through food that grow come from the earth. The best way to get fiber is through food that grows from the earth. The best way to lose weight safely is through eating foods that grow from the earth. The best way to reverse cancer, tumors, diabetes, heart disease, and other illness is by eating food that grows from the earth.

The drug industry has convinced the public to take drugs, dead vitamins, and supplements instead of getting these same vitamins and herbs from eating live, healthy, natural foods. It does not make sense to get dead nutrients from pills, when we can get them naturally from eating live foods. Let's start getting our medicine through natural food. This is the way God has given it to us, so this is the way it should be eaten. When we get our medicine naturally through foods that grow from the earth, we start to feel refreshed, we start to have more energy, and we breathe easier. We start to handle stress better. We start to become, overall, a healthy person.

The Legal Drug World -vs-	**The Illegal Drug World**
1. Pharmaceutical companies give drugs to	1. Drug Lords give illegal drugs to
2. Doctors - who sell the drugs to	2. Drug Sellers who sell the drugs to
3. You - legal drug users	3. Illegal drug users
4. CVS, Eckerd and Walgreen sell these drugs on corners of streets	4. Illegal drug houses sell illegal drugs on corners of streets

Just like the crack addict has to keep going to the crack dealer for more crack many Christians are going to legal drug dealers for their refill of high blood pressure, diabetic, arthritis and cholesterol pills each month. These drugs only cover up symptoms of disease and they never eliminate the primary cause of disease. The only ones to profit are the pharmaceutical companies and the legal drug dealer who sold you the drug and your health never improves. Many of us are no different from illegal drug users.

DID YOU KNOW....?

Proverbs 23:1 When thou sittest to eat, consider diligently what is before thee.

Fast Food

The only food that many people eat is fast food. They eat McDonald's for breakfast, Wendy's for lunch, and Burger King for dinner. This is what people call eating in moderation, but God never intended for us to eat these foods. Almost all food served by these restaurants is fried in greasy fat. This is the same grease that gets into your bloodstream, clogs up your arteries, and causes heart attacks. This is the reason

America's number one killer is heart disease, number two is stroke, and third is cancer. Americans don't even cook anymore. We let fast-food restaurants do the cooking for us, and we are dying from it.

The Meat We Eat

The animals we eat are usually sick and diseased as well before they die. They have cancer, pneumonia, heart disease, and other illnesses due to their environment. They have to breathe in filthy air and drink filthy water, which has their own feces in it. They are kept in small areas with a limited ability to move. From birth, the animals we eat live a life of hell. Heifers that are raised for their milk are pumped with hormones and antibiotics in order for them to produce more milk at a faster rate. These hormones also make the cows grow fast and fat. These hormones are in the cow's milk we feed our children. Remember, the purpose of the hormones and antibiotics is to make cow's grow fat faster and produce milk as fast as possible. We raise our children on cow's milk and now those hormones are making them grow faster and fatter. This is one of the reasons that we have a country full of obese children and adults. We've become a product of our environment.[19,20]

Chickens don't even get to see sunlight. They are raised under artificial lights. Their beaks are cut within days of being born, which mean they aren't able to defend themselves. Studies show that about 98% of all chickens have cancer when they are killed.

Baby bulls, male cows, are raised never to sit or move. Because their diet contains no iron, their meat is white, which is what we call veal. This is the so-called "healthy meat" because it is white. When we eat these diseased animals, it is no wonder they make us sick and diseased. [21,22,23]

When we go to buy meat at the grocery store, we are told the meat is fresh. There is no such thing as fresh meat. The animal is dead so how can it be fresh? Just because it was killed an hour ago doesn't make it fresh. Something that is dead cannot be fresh. Fresh food is live food.

When an animal is killed its meat is not even inspected properly. Less than 1% of all animal products are actually inspected for disease. This means that out of 100 animals killed, only one is inspected for disease.[24,25] Therefore, only one chicken or cow represents the other 99 that were slaughtered, as if the other 99 chickens or cows are disease free. Of those inspected, an inspector has only two seconds per animal to determine if it is diseased.[26] Common sense tells me that is not enough time. The inspector barely has time to get a glimpse of the meat. If a chicken is found to have cancer, the cancerous parts are allowed to be cut out, and the rest of the chicken can be sold for your eating pleasure. Do you think that it is possible for inspectors to miss some of these cancerous spots? If they only have two seconds to look at the meat, I am sure a lot of cancer and other diseases are missed.

Breakfast

Breakfast is a meal that has been over-rated. First, breakfast should not be called break-fast, because it usually is not. Breakfast means the first meal after a fast. A fast is a period of time that a person goes without food. Sleeping at night is not considered a fast. We have been told that breakfast is the most important meal of the day. I am sorry to inform you that I feel this too is incorrect. Let's talk about what the average person eats for breakfast. After a good night's sleep, we awaken to a morning full of energy. After all, sleep is the best way to recharge our bodies to carry on our daily duties. After we wake up full of energy, we kill the energy by eating breakfast. The average breakfast consists of dead foods such as pig, in the form of bacon, sausage or ham; baby chicken embryo in the form of eggs; white bleached bread or flour in the form of pancakes, biscuits, or bagels with butter; mucus-forming sugary syrup, and, to top it off, watered-down sugary flavored fruit juice, or worse, coffee.

Not one of these foods has life in them. The animals are dead, the flour has been bleached and processed, and the drinks are refined sugar and water, not fruit. Now, all that energy we wake up with has to go toward breaking down this dead breakfast we've just eaten. Now you feel sluggish and tired all over again, and it is just the beginning of the morning. How are you going to make it through the rest of the day? This is when drugs like coffee come into play, to help stimulate you and keep you awake. The body does not get any reward, in the form of energy, from breaking this meal down, because the meal has no life. This is how we dig early graves; by eating dead food. After years of abuse, the body is depleted of energy, which leads to sickness and disease. When we wake up feeling refreshed and full of energy, we should use this energy for work or exercise. After work or exercise, we have earned a hunger for food. Reward yourself with life giving foods such as fruit.

Fruit should be eaten first for breakfast, because fruit is the easiest food for the body to digest. It takes the body about 45 minutes to digest fruit and seconds to use it for energy. Fruit also goes through the digestive tract very well, due to high fiber content that cleans out the body along the way. No matter what time your breakfast starts, fruit should be the first food of the day.

If you drink juice, make sure it is freshly squeezed. Juice is not as healthy as most people think. First, it has been taken out of its natural state, which is the fruit or vegetable it is found in. Second, when juicing, we leave out the most important aspect of the fruit or vegetable, which is the fiber. The fiber is needed to clean out the GI tract. Let's use an orange, for example. When we drink a cup of orange juice, it is equal to eating 8 oranges. All this juice can actually be toxic to the body by raising sugar levels. Can we eat 8 oranges at one time? Probably not. After eating two oranges, an apple, and a banana, we will be full. This is how we become allergic to different fruit juices. All this juice was never intended to be in the body at one time. It is healthier for us to eat the whole fruit or vegetable, rather than drink the juice. This way we get juice, fiber, and all the other vitamins and minerals that our body needs. You will never see juice growing from the earth or in trees. Juice is not natural, but fruit and vegetables are.

School Meals

I can recall my high school days when the children would get off the school bus in the morning, and go to the cafeteria to eat breakfast. I enjoyed my breakfast, not knowing at the time it was unhealthy. We were served pig, in the form of bacon and sausage, swimming in grease. The grease would be dripping off the bacon and sausage when I put it in my mouth. We had white processed, buttered bread with jelly on it to make a bacon sandwich. There were never any salads or fruit available, and, if it had been, would I have chosen fruit over a pig? Probably not. To top off my school breakfast, I had sugary watered-down orange or apple juice to drink. There is no way a natural drink can be so sweet. After breakfast, it was time to go to my first period class. I could not concentrate. I would just fall asleep. This is because my body was using all the energy I woke up with to digest the school breakfast I had eaten.

Somehow, I would make it to twelve o'clock - lunchtime. For lunch we may have cows, in the form of hamburger, roast beef or liver; pigs, in the form of ribs or ham; pizza with all kinds of dead animals and grease on it; and our favorite, chicken legs, thighs or breast. Chicken made everyone happy, especially if it was fried. We never ate our vegetables. And to top the meal off, we had cow's milk to drink. Cow's milk is given at every meal in school. You could have your choice of chocolate or white milk. Of course, everyone chose chocolate, because it was sweet. It has two drugs in it, sugar and caffeine. After lunch, the cycle started again. I went to class and fell asleep. My body had to use all the energy that I had to digest the dead foods I had eaten.

These same foods are still given to school children today. High schools now have fast-food restaurants in them, so if children don't want the cafeteria food they can buy junk food. Schools also have soft drink machines on every corner now. Schools today seldom serve healthy food to our children, and if they do, the children probably don't eat it.

With the diet and drugs we are feeding our school kids, it is no wonder our children are overweight, have ADD (Attention Deficit Disorder), and ADHD (Attention Deficit Hyperactivity Disorder). It is no wonder our kids are prone to diabetes, cancer, heart disease, stroke, etc.

Hospitals and Doctors

Not only are children being fed dead food in schools, patients are being fed dead food in hospitals. A hospital is a place where we should recover from sickness, but the foods served in hospitals can prolong your recovery, or even kill you. I can remember working for a children's hospital where every minute a child would come into the hospital with a cold, flu, head and stomach aches. These children would be given a shot or medicine to cover up the symptoms, and they would leave with a soda, chewing gum, or ice-cream in their hands or candy in their mouths. They were given the same foods that probably caused the illness to begin with. I recall visiting an aunt in a hospital who had suffered a stroke. At her dinner meal, she was given cow's milk and tea, chicken, a white dough ball called a roll, and some jell-O. The only healthy thing on her plate was broccoli, and it was covered in cheese. I remember my aunt asking my mother if she should be eating that type of food. My mom replied, "Well, since the hospital serves the food, then it must be good for you. After all, the doctors know what is best for you." This is how many people think. If the doctor says it is healthy, then it must be. This is far from the truth.

You cannot restore health quickly by eating dead foods. The best way to restore your health safely and quickly is to eat live foods. Most importantly, the best way to prevent disease is to eat a majority of God's Original Diet and live a healthy lifestyle. I don't want anyone to think that I am against hospitals. I know they are needed, especially emergency rooms. The greatest doctors in the world are emergency room physicians because they save lives everyday. If you are in an emergency life-threatening situation, the hospital is for you. I don't think that hospitals are the best place to go for long-term health care. Doctors that spend their time writing out medicine prescriptions for their patients all day don't help their patients.

These types of doctors are not getting to the primary cause of their patients' problems. They are only covering up symptoms. The word doctor means to teach. It is time for doctors to teach their patients why they are suffering from the diseases they have. It is time for doctors to teach their patients how they can prevent disease instead of telling them to take a pill to cover up symptoms of the disease. Doctors should teach their patients why they are overweight and teach them how to lose weight safely, instead of offering them surgeries and weight loss pills. Surgeries, weight loss pills, and medicine don't get to the primary cause of sickness, they only cover up symptoms. When a person gets sick, most doctors cannot tell them how they got sick, because they don't know. Nutrition is not taught properly in medical schools. Nutrition is taught the way man wants to teach it - "The Four Basic Food Groups" - and not the way God said we should eat.

It amazes me that man has the knowledge to cut out different organs that have cancer, tumors, and other diseases, but doesn't have a clue how the patient got the disease in the first place. Doctors can cut out cancerous intestines, kidneys, ovaries, and other organs, but cannot tell the patient where the cancer came from. I have seen surgeons cut out cancerous organs and afterwards go and eat a pizza or hamburger with greasy French fries. This tells me that they have no clue how diseases come about. Most are only taught to treat the disease after it enters the body, instead of teaching the patient how to prevent the disease in the first place.

The original fast food is the food God made for man to eat. Eating fruits, vegetables, raw nuts, seeds, and whole grains is healthy for the body. These foods don't have to be cooked. God has given them flavor and all the nutrients man needs to be healthy. All we have to do is eat them, and they will give us energy and life, not sickness and disease.

If you want to loose weight in a healthy way, prevent diseases, have energy, and breathe easier, you can do so by eating a majority of God's Original Diet. When you eat these foods, you can eat all you want until you are full and satisfied, and you will still lose the weight you desire in a healthy way.

When you start to eat the way God intended, diseases go away, energy comes into the body, stress is handled better, you have a positive outlook on life, rest comes easier, and you have an overall healthier body. This is what God intended for His children. God never intended for His children to be sick, diseased, and in poor health. God never intended for His children to take medicine everyday, to give all their hard earned money to doctors, or to do every diet fad that comes around. God wants His people to be in perfect health. Humans have gotten away from the way God instructed us to eat, and we are suffering sickness and disease because of it. Humans are the only animals that get sick because you will not find animals in nature suffering with headaches, diabetes, high blood pressure, cancer, and obesity. Sure, your pet may get sick, but that's because the pet eats like the owner. Humans are the only animals that don't live out their normal lifespan. Dogs and cats in the wild live ten to twelve years, their normal lifespan. Monkeys, horses, camels, and elephants can live to be fifty to a hundred years old, their normal lifespan. Humans' normal lifespan, according to science, and most importantly God, in Genesis chapter 6, verse 3, is one-hundred and twenty years, but most only live half of that. We lose half our lifespan because we disobey God's natural laws of health. It was never God's will for His children to be sick. Sickness is not of God.

St. John 10:10 states "I come that they might have life, and that they might have it more abundantly."

III.
Feed Me With Food Convenient For Me

In the Name of Weight Loss

During the New Year's holiday, I love to spend time with my family. It is a time when we can look back and talk about old times. We talk about the blessings that God has bestowed upon us and thank Him. My family, like every family, makes resolutions for the New Year. Losing weight is on top of everyone's list of New Year's resolutions. They eat a big meal on January 1st, and decide to go on a diet afterwards. They begin to workout, run, and lift weights and begin to eat foods they think are healthy. When the end of January rolls around and no weight has been lost, they become discouraged and stop.

People stop dieting and exercising from February to December, and when the next year rolls around, the same resolutions are made and the same cycle is repeated. These new-year-resolution diets never work permanently, and most of the time they're not healthy. My family members see a friend losing weight very quickly on a particular diet and they want to try it themselves. A month later the person is bigger than they were before they started the diet. This happens every year, and nothing is ever accomplished. I am sure there are other families like this. We only diet when we want to fit into a swimsuit during the summer, go to a high school or college reunion or other events where our bodies will be exposed. These events motivate us to loose weight so people will not talk about us. If you eat healthy all year, you won't have to worry about losing weight when these events come around because you would already be at your desired weight. It should not take a New Year or reunion to motivate us to get healthy.

Americans spend billions of dollars a year on weight loss programs, weight loss pills, and surgeries. If we are spending all this money, why is over half the population fat or obese? We are looking at genes, bugs, the environment, heredity, and other causes for obesity. The answer is not found there. The answer is found in how we eat and live. We all know that if you eat an excessive amount of food, then you will get fat, right? This may or may not be true. The type of food we eat can also make a difference in determining our weight. Almost all diets are based on false information. We watch television commercials that show obese people who, after one month on a diet program, are in great shape, without ever changing their lifestyle.

There is no way to loose weight permanently and in a healthy way without changing our eating and living habits. Most diets don't focus on permanent weight loss and permanent health. The only way any diet will work permanently, is if it is something a person can live with for the rest of their life. There are many things people do to lose weight, and many can be life threatening. Many people have lost their lives trying to lose weight. They may have taken a pill or they may have had parts of their body surgically removed. There are many weight loss pills that claim they can help you lose weight, and chances are they have some side effects. Weight loss pills will help you lose weight, but you may lose your life in the process. If you are blessed to not lose your life, you may end up with life-long health problems. Pills like Fen-phen, that can cause heart problems, are not worth taking just to lose weight.[1]

People also have surgery to help them lose weight. People have had parts of their small intestines removed, fat sucked out of their abdomen, and some have had their stomachs stapled to lose weight. God did not intend man to staple his stomach. God did not give man organs to remove, except in life or death situations. Obesity is not an emergency situation. All of our organs play important roles in survival, and when we take them out, it lessens our survival rate.

You cannot lose weight *healthily* just by drinking a shake everyday. You cannot lose weight *healthily* by taking a pill, and you surely cannot find healthy weight loss in surgeries. You will loose weight with most diets, but the majority are not healthy. The only healthy diet is God's Original Diet. With this diet we can eat until we are full, never depriving ourselves of a variety of good food.

Man-made Diets Do Not Work

> *Proverbs 23:2 And put a knife to thy throat, if thou be a man given to appetite.*

Let's discuss some popular diets. The high protein and low carbohydrate diets are probably the craziest diets I have ever heard of. Many people love these diets, because it's just what they want to hear. Most people are amazed to hear that they can eat all the meat they want, and lose weight. The Atkins and Zone diets have nothing to do with health, only weight loss. You will lose weight on these diets, along with your health. They can be very dangerous, and they have many side effects. Think about it; eliminate most of the foods God gave us, and eat only man-made foods. You can eat all the dead pigs, cows, and chickens you want, and still lose weight.

The weight lost on these diets is water weight. When we go on a diet, we do not want to lose water, we want to lose fat. After all, our bodies are made up of 75% water, which means that we are mostly water. And water is life. When we loose water, we are losing a part of ourselves. The body uses water to aid in the digestion of food. If we do not put water into our bodies by drinking it or eating healthy foods, the body uses the water that it already has stored to aid in digestion. This means that if we eat mostly meats, our body has to use stored water to digest the meat. After eating meat for a long period of time, you will lose weight - water weight - not fat.[2] Water is life, and to lose it causes sickness and disease. In fact, one of the side effects from a heavy meat diet is dehydration, because, again, the body has to use stored water to digest the meat. Other side effects are constipation and fatigue; because meat has no fiber, it just sits in the intestines.[3] Think about what happens to our bodies when we eat mostly meat - we have no energy and no life.

Diseases such as cancer, arthritis, and heart disease occur with these diets.[4,5,6] Eating meats with high saturated fat clogs up the arteries, so people on these diets may have high blood pressure and atherosclerosis, which can lead to a heart attack or stroke.[7,8] These diets also cause people to have high blood cholesterol, because meat and dairy products are the only foods that contain cholesterol.[9] Protein from meat can harden in the blood and, with the calcium that is used to break it down, can form stones in the kidneys and gallbladder.[10] These diets also recommend that you take vitamins and even have diet candy bars you can eat. If you have to take vitamins and eat candy bars to make up for nutrients you're not getting, then the diet is not healthy. The authors of these famous diets do not appear to be healthy and, in my view, appear to be overweight themselves. One even had heart problems before his death, so who are they to give advice on losing weight.

Eliminating God's original foods from your diet can be very dangerous to your health, so it only makes sense to include a majority of them in your diet. These are the only foods that provide your body with energy and health, and they allow you to lose weight in the process.

Now let's talk about the low carbohydrate diet. This diet says that people should eliminate carbohydrates to lose weight. It also says that if you crave carbohydrates, then you are addicted to them, as if carbohydrates are a type of drug. Carbohydrates are not drugs. I can just imagine a carbohydrate addict, walking around obsessing for a carbohydrate. Eliminating carbohydrates from your diet will cause weight loss, but not healthy weight loss. Carbohydrates are essential nutrients needed in our diet. It is the source of the carbohydrates we eat that causes weight gain. If we get our carbohydrates from processed cereals, white refined pastas, white refined breads and bagels, white rice, dairy products, donuts etc., then we can expect to gain weight, because these foods have no life in them. It is not the carbohydrates you are addicted to, it is chemicals and drugs that are put in these foods that you are addicted to.

Just because you eat unhealthy foods with carbohydrates in them, does not mean that you are addicted to the carbohydrates. It is the types of food that these carbohydrates are in that you are addicted to. Eliminate these foods from your diet, not carbohydrates. Eliminating fruits and vegetables from your diet just because they contain carbohydrates can be very dangerous. Along with the unhealthy weight loss, you will be constipated and experience a loss of energy. This is because you are not eating live foods and foods that contain fiber. Don't eliminate carbohydrates from your diet; eliminate processed and refined foods from your diet.

Carbohydrates are found in many healthy foods such as wheat, oats, legumes, fruits, and vegetables. Start eating a majority of these foods and watch your weight drop and your energy rise. There is only one diet that allows you to eat all the foods you want for the rest of your life and be healthy at the same time. This diet is called, God's Original Diet.

IV.
For They Are Deceitful Meat (Food)

There are many foods that we have been brainwashed to believe are healthy, but they are not. If we look at the four basic food groups, on which our nation is based, we find that 75% consists of dead foods. The food guide pyramid, which is a guide to daily food choices, tells us to eat 6 to 11 servings of the bread, cereal, rice, and pasta group and 2 to 3 servings of the meat, poultry, fish, eggs, dry beans, and nuts group. It says we should eat 2 to 3 servings from the milk, yogurt, and cheese group. Last, we should include 3 to 5 servings of vegetables and 2 to 4 servings of fruit.

Man's Diet

First of all, I don't understand the word "serving", because that is too complex for me. It is similar to counting calories. I don't understand it and don't want to understand it. When I sit at the dinner table, I like to eat and not think about how many calories and servings I'm eating. I like to eat until I am full and when that happens I stop eating, not caring about how many calories I have eaten and if I ate the right amount of servings.

Following the four-basic-food-groups is a man-made diet. With this diet man has eaten himself into many diseases. God has already told us the diet to eat in Genesis 1:29. The original four basic food groups were fruits, vegetables, raw nuts and seeds, and whole grains.

Man's diet consists of 75% dead foods. God's original diet consists of 100% live foods. Man's diet causes obesity and fatigue. God's original diet will shed pounds and give energy. Man's diet causes sickness and disease. God's Original Diet gives life and life more abundantly. God knows what is best for His children.

The foods described on the following pages are man-made and don't contain the nutrients your body needs. If you want to be healthy, learn how these dead foods affect you and begin to reduce or eliminate them from your diet.

Coffee

Coffee is one of many legal drugs. Coffee is addictive, and like all illegal drugs, it is hard for a person to give it up once they are addicted to it. Coffee with sugar contains two legal drugs - caffeine and sugar. Many people drink coffee every morning to help them wake up. If you need coffee to wake up in the morning, or for a quick energy burst, then you are probably addicted to it. Coffee stimulates the nervous system and gives a sensation of energy. Over time this can be very detrimental towards a person's health. Coffee makes a person hyper, or full of energy, which is false energy because the body gets no energy in return for getting rid of it. Coffee takes a high percentage of calcium out of bones to neutralize the pH level in our blood, which can lead to osteoporosis.[1]

Coffee keeps you from getting proper sleep because it is a stimulant.[2] Coffee addicts who try to break the coffee habit experience the same symptoms that a crack addict goes through when they wean themselves off crack. People tell me all the time if they don't drink coffee they will get a headache. As soon as they drink coffee the headache goes away. They begin to believe that they need coffee to take away their headaches, but actually, it is coffee that is causing the headaches. This is the body's way of getting rid of the toxins. Headaches are one of the symptoms a person must endure for drinking coffee.[3]

The body gets rid of coffee through the kidneys, which actually puts stress on the kidneys. Have you ever noticed how much you urinate when you drink coffee? The body has to use water already in the body to get rid of coffee. This means that good water, already in the body, is used to flush the coffee out. This is the body's way of saying, "I do not want this toxic chemical in me, so I will use the good water that I already have to get rid of it." We drink one cup of coffee, and pee out two cups. This makes us feel dehydrated because the body has to eliminate valuable water from the body. The kidneys' job is to filter the blood. The foods we eat and drink determine how hard the kidneys will work. The kidneys were never designed to filter out drugs like coffee. Years of abusing caffeine, along with other various drugs, can cause problems with the kidneys. If you are addicted to this drug, start to wean yourself off of it today. You will suffer from withdrawal symptoms for a short period of time, but when it is over you will feel great.

Sodas

Sodas are legal drugs. They also contain the drugs caffeine and sugar. The body processes soda the same way it processes coffee. We drink one can of soda and pee out two cans of liquid. The body has to get rid of it, because it is poison to the systems of the body. Sodas, like coffee, make the kidneys work very hard and eventually, over time after abusing these legal drugs, they may shut down. Sodas also take calcium out of bones, due to the calcium/phosphorus ratio. The body should have a 2:1 calcium to phosphorus ratio. Sodas have lots of phosphorus in them and phosphorus is a mineral found in bones and blood. When the body has too much phosphorus in the blood, the body will take calcium from the bones to help balance the ratio. When we drink sodas in excessive amounts, the body has to keep taking calcium out of bones to keep the ratio balanced. Calcium taken out of bone in excessive amounts will eventually lead to osteoporosis.

There is one advantage to having a Coke around. If battery acid is building up around your battery cables in your vehicle, you can pour Coke on them, and within minutes the acid around the battery cables will dissolve. Coke will dissolve battery acid and every car mechanic knows this. If sodas dissolve battery acid, imagine what it can do to the stomach, kidneys, and other organs. The sulfuric acid from sodas burns your throat when you try to swallow it. No wonder people go on dialysis and need kidney transplants. There is no such thing as a healthy soda, no matter the color.

Tobacco

Tobacco found in cigars, snuff, cigarettes, and other legal drugs is one of the major killers in our society. More people die of cancer from smoking tobacco than any other legal or illegal drugs. Cigarette and cigar companies make millions of dollars a year and kill hundreds of thousands in the process.[32] They figure that if they put the warning signs at the bottom of each carton, then it is up to you to take that chance with your life. In a way, this may be true. Even though people know cigarettes are bad for them, many choose to smoke anyway. Most children begin smoking just to fit in with the crowd. They figure they will smoke while they are teens and quit when they become adults. When these children become adults, and try to quit smoking, they find it very hard to do. Their plan to quit when they become an adult fails because, as teenagers, we don't realize that cigarettes are drugs. The cigarette companies know this is going to happen, before you even attempt to smoke your first cigarette. They know that once a child starts to smoke at a young age, it is hard for them to quit later in life. This means you make the cigarette companies richer and you die slowly. You are paying them to kill you.

Cigarette smoking is advertised as the cool thing to do. It makes you look pretty. It keeps women slim, trim, and sexy. It makes the male seem manly. Children are the main targets for tobacco advertising, and many parents are so busy today they don't have time to teach their kids the important lessons in life.[33] This is when the television, gangs, and drug dealers began to teach our kids, and when our kids get in trouble we wonder why it happened. Most advertising targets children, because children are easily persuaded.

Cigarette companies may tell you, the parent, that your child should wait until he is 18 to smoke, but can you trust them? Advertising shows what appears to be a "cool life" if you smoke. They show that you can have a fun life if you smoke. What they don't show is the end of that life, after smoking. They don't show the cancer that forms after years of smoking. They don't show parts of the lung that have to be taken out because of smoking. They do not show how the larynx has to be taken out because cancer from smoking has destroyed it, and now the person cannot talk. They do not show how difficult it is for a person to breathe because his lungs are over inflated with the disease emphysema. They do not show the person who has to struggle for every ounce of air in order to breathe and stay alive. They do not show you that eventually, that cool person may eventually die from a smoking-related disease. Cigarette companies know that smoking eventually leads to death, but do you think they care about your life? Probably not. Cigarettes are more addictive than marijuana, heroin, alcohol, or any other legal or illegal drugs.

Tobacco has a drug in it called nicotine, and it is a very addictive poison. Nicotine causes confusion, muscular twitching, cramps, convulsions, depression, central nervous system paralysis, respiratory failure, and other major symptoms. Nicotine is also used as an insecticide to kill different insects that destroy crops. Nicotine is so dangerous that only small amounts can be put in cigarettes, or it would kill you. If you inhaled the nicotine found in one pack of cigarettes all at one time, it would be enough to kill you instantly.[34,35] With every puff you take from a cigarette, you are shortening your days, and allowing your body to be taken over with sickness and disease.

Cigarette smoke contains more than just the poison nicotine; there are thousands of chemicals found in cigarette smoke. Cigarette smoke contains carbon monoxide - a toxic gas found in car exhaust; formaldehyde - a toxic gas used to preserve dead bodies; and ammonia - chemical compound of nitrogen and hydrogen used to make bombs, toilet bowl, and floor cleaners. It is believed that there are over 4,000 harmful or deadly chemicals found in cigarette smoke.[36] It is no wonder smoking is one of the leading causes of cancer. After breathing in over 4,000 chemicals a day, it is a wonder that smokers' bodies last as long as they do.

Smoking contributes to the top three killers in our society, which are heart disease, cancer, and stroke. Other illness and disease that smoking has been linked to are emphysema, bronchitis, ulcers, osteoporosis, abortions, fetal death and birth defects of newborns, cataracts, impotence, infertility, destruction of the mucus membranes that line the GI tract, and destruction of cells.[37,38] Smoking also leaves your lips and fingers very dirty and dark, which is caused by the destruction of the cells in the lips and fingers. Smokers use more seasoning on their food, such as salt, pepper, and hot sauces because the smoke slowly destroys their taste buds. It is estimated that starting to smoke in the late teens will reduce life expectancy by an average of 9 or more years. Breast cancer is found at a 75% higher rate in women who smoke. Smoking is linked to cancers of the mouth, larynx, esophagus, urinary tract, kidneys, pancreas, and cervix.[39] Children who suffer from allergies, asthma, and other lung illnesses usually have parents who smoke.

Smoking during pregnancy is linked to bleeding, miscarriage, premature delivery, lower birth weight, and sudden infant death syndrome (SIDS).[40] Studies now show that secondhand smoke is worse than first-hand smoke. Secondhand smoke can kill nonsmokers faster than first-hand smoke kills smokers. Secondhand smoke contains nicotine, tar, carbon monoxide, and other harmful chemicals, just as first-hand smoke does. Secondhand smoke speeds up the heart rate and destroys blood vessels, which raises blood pressure and doubles the carbon monoxide in your blood. This means that not only do smokers kill themselves, but may kill others in the process.[41]

And let's not forget the little things smoking does. Smoking makes your clothes and breath smell bad and leaves tar stains on your teeth that no toothpaste can remove.

There is nothing sadder than to see someone coughing because they cannot get an adequate supply of air. It is sad to see friends and family die of something that they could have prevented. Every adult knows that smoking is bad for them, even before they take their first puff. I have had many friends and family members die because of this cigarette drug, and I will probably see many more die if they do not stop smoking. Sadly, doctors have told my family members that, after smoking thirty to fifty years, cigarettes did not contribute to their cancer. They were told their cancer was genetic. Statements like this show how ignorant some doctors are, even when it comes to cigarettes. I cannot state this clearly enough - cigarettes cause cancer. If it were not for cigarettes, lung cancer would be almost nonexistent. When you die cigarette companies don't care. They are happy to take your money, and you pay for cigarettes with your life.

If you are a smoker, try to stop today. I understand it is easier said than done, but I am amazed how easy it is to quit smoking after the doctor tells you that you have lung cancer and you only have a short time to live. Most people get the willpower to quit when they hear those words, but then it is usually too late. Don't let a death sentence give you the willpower to quit; please quit before you hear those words. A person cannot quit until they make up their own mind that they want to. You have to want to quit for yourself and not for your spouse, children, or anyone else.

Alcohol

Alcohol can impair your thinking and your vision as well as motor activities such as driving and walking. Alcohol causes liver and kidney disease, and damages the brain and heart. Alcohol can cause fetal alcohol syndrome and it increases your risk for cancer.[14,15] It is a legal drug that is very addictive. For years people have been told that red wine is a healthy food. We are told that red wine helps the heart and helps lower cholesterol.

They do not tell about the liver damage alcohol causes. Cirrhosis of the liver is most commonly caused by alcohol intake. Alcohol is very toxic to the liver, and it interferes with glucose getting to the brain, causing the brain to malfunction. This causes the staggering, impaired speech, and depression often seen in people drinking alcohol. Alcohol is so poisonous that it causes brain tissue loss. Alcohol also contributes to malnutrition, because most alcoholics have no desire for food. Alcohol impairs calcium absorption in the bones by stopping the liver from making vitamin D. Vitamin D is important for helping put calcium into bone. The more alcohol you drink, the less your body is able to put calcium into bones, leading to osteoporosis. Alcohol may cause cancer of the mouth, pharynx, larynx, and esophagus.

Red wine is not a healthy drink, but juice from red grapes is. It is not red wine that helps the heart, it is red grapes. It is not red wine that lowers cholesterol, it is the juice of red grapes. There is nothing that red wine can do that red grape juice can't do better. Red grapes work better before they are made into wine. Every healthy nutrient found in red wine is also found in red grapes. Alcohol contains no nutrients that the body needs. Instead of drinking red wine, just eat red grapes and forget the alcohol. Red grapes alone will give the benefits that so-called health experts have attributed to red wine. If you are a person that drinks alcohol, start eliminating it from your diet today.

> *Proverbs 20:1 Wine is a mocker, strong drink is raging: and whosoever is deceived thereby is not wise.*

Kool-aid and Fruit Juices

Kool-aid is a childhood favorite. Kool-aid is mostly sugar, water, and dye. We see commercials on television with little kids showing their Kool-aid smiles. They tell us that it has vitamin C added and that makes it good for children. The commercials should show the smile when the kids are teenagers, with a mouth full of cavities and missing teeth. When you spill Kool-aid on a countertop, desk, or clothes, it stains them. Washing the clothes or using S.O.S. pads on stained surfaces often will not remove the stains. If the dyes in Kool-aid put stains on countertops and clothes, imagine what it does to your stomach. These dyes can stain the lining of the GI tract and affect the absorption of nutrients into the bloodstream.

Fruit juices are very popular, but are these drinks really made of fruit? In most cases they are not. There are a lot of artificially-flavored fruit drinks on the market. There are a lot of drinks that say they are made of real fruit, but are really made of artificially-flavored fruit, sugar, and water. This means that they are the same as Kool-aid. They have no nutritional value. If you look at the nutritional label on these drinks, you will see they contain little real fruit juice.

These drinks say that vitamin C is added, but why should vitamin C be added, when it is already found in the real fruit juice? Some symptoms of drinking these fruit juices are low back pain, headaches, cavities, colds, and diabetes. The healthiest fruit juice is freshly squeezed fruit juice. These juices help build up your immune system to fight off various diseases.

Cow's Milk

We cannot drive down a major highway or watch a program on television without seeing a celebrity drinking a glass of cow's milk with a milk mustache. Sure, cow's milk has calcium, but it is not the best source for humans. Your body prefers calcium from plants, nuts, seeds, and grains over the calcium found in cow's milk. Cow's milk is high in cholesterol, fat, hormones, antibiotics, glue, and pus. Cow's milk has 400% more calcium, 15% more protein , and more phosphorus than human milk. This is to support the calf's faster growth rate. Human milk has 5 to 7% protein, to support our slow growth rate.[5] Humans cannot use the calcium, proteins, and phosphorus found in cow's milk because we are not calves. Human milk has 6 to 10 times the essential fatty acids than cow's milk. Cows have four stomachs to digest their milk and humans only have one stomach to digest milk and other foods.

Humans who drink 3 to 4 glasses of cow's milk each day increase their secondary sex characteristics - larger breast, early menstruation, and the ability to reproduce. The same protein used to make glue, casein, is found at levels 20 times higher in cow's milk than mother's milk. This makes cow's milk very difficult for humans to digest and absorb.[6]

Cow's milk is so unhealthy, that it has to be pasteurized before consumption because of the contaminants it contains. Pasteurization kills both good and bad bacteria. Milk should be drunk raw, not pasteurized. All animals feed their babies raw milk. You will never see a cow heating her milk and then feeding it to her calf; she feeds the calf raw milk. You will never see a dog feeding her puppies pasteurized milk; dogs give their puppies raw milk. Raw milk is live milk. When we pasteurize and heat milk we kill it. Mothers that breastfeed their infants do not heat and pasteurize their milk. When you pasteurize and heat milk, you kill all the hormones and the antibodies that the infant needs in order to grow and fight off diseases. Start to give your newborn mother's milk because it is the best milk you can give your child.[7]

Humans are the only animals that drink milk as adults, and the only animals that drink another animal species' milk. No other animal in nature drinks cow's milk but calves. All animals in nature drink their own species' milk, and after the baby stage, they are weaned off milk and drink only water the rest of their lives. Humans should do the same. Cow's milk is not a health food. Don't be fooled by information the dairy industry gives us about cow's milk being healthy. Low fat milk is actually high in fat; it still contains 24-33% fat. Two percent (2%) milk still has 35% fat in it. It is 2% fat only by it's weight, with extra water. If you "got milk," you may have other illness to go along with it. If you suffer with obesity, allergies, heart disease, colic, muscle cramps, sinusitis, skin rashes, acne, GI bleeding, diarrhea, iron deficiency anemia, arthritis, ear infections, asthma, diabetes, cataracts, osteoporosis, a host of cancers, and multiple sclerosis, cows milk could be playing a role.[8,9,10,11,12,13] This is not a health food; this is a dead food. Eliminate it from your diet today.

Eggs

Eggs are one of America's favorite foods. Breakfast is not complete without eggs. We are told that eggs are our best source of protein. Eggs are not even considered meat. Eggs consist of a chicken embryo, placenta, and a shell to protect the embryo. When we eat eggs, we are eating the fetus and placenta of a baby chicken and, seasoned with a little salt and pepper, chicken fetus is tasty. You can fry it or scramble it. Eggs, like all dairy products, are high in cholesterol, saturated fat, have no fiber, and increase your risk for disease.[16] This sounds like a food that health experts would tell you not to eat. Your body does not gain any benefit from eating eggs, and many people bloat and have stomach cramps after eating them. This is your body's way of telling you that it cannot use this food.

Chickens are fed hormones, antibiotics, arsenic, and other harmful chemicals to stimulate growth and kill parasites.[17] These same chemicals are passed to the fetus in the egg, and when we eat an egg, we are also ingesting these chemicals. Eggs are not a health food and they should be reduced in your diet.

Margarine

Margarine was created when butter was rare and America was trying to cut down on its cholesterol intake. Margarine is made from vegetable oils and other chemicals and has a butter-like taste. Of course, if it comes from vegetable oils it has to be healthy right? Wrong. These vegetable oils go through a process called hydrogenation, where the oils are heated above their boiling point. The vegetable oils go from a cis fat to a trans fat that our bodies cannot use, meaning it has the same makeup as saturated fat.

Margarine has so much hydrogen added to it that it turns into a solid grease stick. Margarine clogs up arteries with fat, and enough of it can contribute to heart attacks and strokes.[18] If you are eating margarine, start to reduce it or eliminate it from your diet.

Nut Butters

Nut butters found in most grocery stores are not digestible by the body. Name-brand nut butters are big business with children and adults. I know this is a healthy food, but, of course, man has a way to make it unhealthy. Peanut and other butters found in most grocery stores are not good for the body. These butters go through a heating process and have hydrogen atoms added to them, the same as margarine. These butters also have salt, sugars, and other chemicals added to them to enhance flavor. The fats found in them are trans fatty acids, which has the same makeup as saturated fat. Excessive amounts of these fats clog up the arteries feeding the heart and brain. Have you noticed that the oils found in name-brand peanut butters are always in the mixture of the peanut butter when you open the jar? These oils are so heavy that they cannot rise to the top of the butter.

Naturally ground peanut butter oils stay above the butter. The fat found in naturally ground peanut butter is cis fat. Oils that have been heated and processed remain within the mixture of the butter. There are many naturally-ground nut butters that you can buy such as peanut, almonds, cashews, and many more.

Sugar

Sugar is a drug used to sweeten different foods. Sugar is usually made from beets or cane, and it makes up a large percentage of the American diet. We have sugar in our drinks, all desserts, and even kids' cereals. When sugar is processed, all the minerals, vitamins, fiber, enzymes, and other nutrients are destroyed. This leaves a dead chemical for the body to digest, providing the body with no energy in return for digesting it. Sugar is put in foods to make people crave it. Cakes, pies, sweet drinks, and all sweet foods can be addictive.

Sometimes parents bribe kids, telling them that they will not get desert if they do not eat their vegetables. When kids cry in church, we stuff candy or gum in their mouths to keep them quiet. When we want kids to do a chore, we reward them with sugary sweets. Sugar is not a healthy food and it deprives the brain of its proper sugar, called glucose.[19]

Excess sugar deprives the brain of energy, and can cause a person to act out or become confused. This is called a sugar high or rush. When a person has a sugar high his/her brain is depleted of glucose and the sugar clouds the brain. This causes the person to be irritable and have an ill temper. As soon as the body can fight off the sugar, the person is back to their normal self. Does this sound like a drug to you? These are some of the same symptoms found with kids suffering from ADD and hyperactivity. Many doctors think that ADD comes from dysfunctions of the mind, and this may be true. But, it could be something as simple as sugar and other dead foods feeding the brain that are making our kids act the way they do today.[20] Sugar irritates the digestive organs and affects the brain just like any other drug.

Sugar takes away the desire for nutritious foods because it is so addictive. When excess sugar is added to our diet, we start to lose the body's demand to store vitamins, minerals, and other nutrients. Our bodies become deficient in these important minerals because of our sugar addiction. This can lead to vitamin deficiency diseases, diabetes, cavities, etc.[21]

Sugar may satisfy your sweet tooth, but in the long run it can cause that same sweet tooth to form cavities. The best sugar for the body is the sugar found in fruits and vegetables. These are the sugars that God has made for man to eat.

Salt

Salt is a very addictive drug that is contributing to the decline of Americans' health everyday. Salt adds flavor to every food imaginable. Salt is put in dairy products, canned goods, refined and processed breads, potato chips, and even baby foods.

Salt is one of the most addictive drugs we eat, and it is poison to the body. The body has to get rid of it as soon as it enters the body. Salt absorbs water like a sponge. Have you ever noticed how thirsty you get when you eat salty foods? When you eat ice cream, potato chips, salty buttered popcorn, and even when you drink sodas, you get thirsty.

This is because these foods have high salt contents. When large amounts of salt enter the body, it triggers the thirst center in the brain to drink. Water will flush the salt out of the body through urine. Salt robs the body of water which, makes us thirsty

35

after consuming salty meals and drinks. Salt is a magnet to water, which means where salt is, water will follow. When there is excess salt in the diet, the body has to get rid of it. The body's favorite place to put salt is in the lower extremities - knees and ankles. Salt is also stored in the lower portion of the GI tract, eyelids, and jaws.[22] When the body puts excess salt in the ankles, water must follow.

The body sends water with salt in it to help dilute the tissues surrounding joints. This is a protective mechanism the body uses so that salt will not destroy the surrounding tissue. This causes swollen ankles, puffy eyelids, and obesity. I can recall in my childhood years, that when my dad was ready to sell a cow, he would always feed it salt. We had a salt block in our pasture and the cows loved to lick it. After the cows licked the salt block, they would immediately run to the pond for water to drink. The salt would make them thirsty, and after the cow filled up on water it would be taken to the sale barn and weighed on a scale. The cow, full of water, would weigh much more and my dad made more money. The same is true with the obesity problem that America faces today. Salt is only one of many factors that contribute to the overweight problems we are fighting. Salt is not a healthy food, but rather a drug. Salt robs the body of nutrients, and when salt is eaten in excess, it can lead to osteoporosis, high blood pressure, obesity, kidney damage, cancers, cardiovascular disease, and much more.[23,24,25]

Start eating organic salts found in foods that grow from the earth. All foods that grow from the earth have traces of salt in them. This is the same amount of salt that our bodies need; only small amounts. Foods that grow from the earth provide the body with the necessary amounts of nutrients, including organic salt. Foods like green leafy vegetables, celery, nuts, and beans provide the body with the necessary amount of organic sodium the body needs to survive. Your body would prefer the sodium from the earth, rather than the table salt from man. Give your body the sodium it deserves for healthy living.

Fried Foods

There is hardly any food that people cannot find a way to fry. As long as we have some oil and meal, we can find a way to fry food. We fry vegetables, meats, and even fruit. When vegetables are fried, the oil is heated over its boiling point. This causes the oil to harden, and makes it very hard for the body to digest. These heated oils, just like animal fats, clog up arteries and cause other health-related problems.

These same fats get into our bloodstream and harden our arteries, especially the arteries that supply blood to the heart and brain. When arteries are clogged we suffer from high blood pressure, which will eventually lead to heart attacks and strokes. It is no wonder two of America's top three killers are heart disease and stroke. The body tries to get rid of fried foods immediately, but this is sometimes hard to do if we eat foods that don't contain fiber. The fried food just sits in our stomach and begins to secrete poisons, which can lead to obesity, cancer, arthritis, tumors, stone formation, and other illnesses.

Processed Refined Foods

Processed refined foods such as white rice, white bread, bagels, donuts, pasta, flour, sugar, etc. are common foods consumed everyday. Most breakfast food consists of white bread toast, bagels, biscuits, pancakes or white rice. Lunch consists of sandwiches made of white processed breads and dinner consists of bleached cornbread, white flour bread, and sweets made of processed, refined flours. Even major restaurants have pasta listed as a vegetable, and they are in the same section with the real vegetables. Macaroni and spaghetti aren't vegetables; they are lifeless pasta, and pasta means paste.

Processing takes the nutrients out of foods. Let's take white rice, for example. When rice is harvested from the earth, it contains nutrients the body needs. Rice is brown when it contains these nutrients and is brown when it is harvested. Man takes this perfect food and bleaches it, destroying valuable nutrients. When rice is bleached, vitamins, minerals, fiber, and other important nutrients are destroyed in the process. The food is literally killed, and chemicals are added to enhance the appearance of the food, texture, and flavor. All unrefined foods have the same basic structure - they have a single grain, which is the seed; an outer coating, which is the bran or fiber layer; an inner layer, which is the endosperm; and the lower portion of the inner layer, which is the germ. The bran layer is the outer coating of the seed which is used for protection until the seed germinates. The germ is the life of the seed, containing oils, vitamins, and a variety of minerals, proteins, and carbohydrates. The endosperm is part of the germ layer that draws nutrients from the soil, but all the nutrients are collected in the germ layer. In the process of refining these foods the bran layer is removed - there goes the fiber. Next, the germ from the germ layer is removed - there go all the vitamins, minerals proteins, and the rest of the nutrients in the food.

Removing the germ and the fiber defeats the purpose of eating food. The purpose of eating food is to provide our body with nutrients, and then we eliminate them through the bowels with the help of fiber. To get this benefit, the food needs to contain nutrients and fiber. Processing foods removes nutrients and fiber. The only thing left after processing is the endosperm, which is a starchy product of the food. The endosperm has no life, and the original food is destroyed. The endosperm, however, is non-perishable, meaning that it will not spoil. The main purpose for processing food is to allow a longer shelf life for the food. White rice will last longer on your shelves than brown rice. White bread will last longer on your shelves than wheat or rye bread. Any processed, bleached food will have a longer shelf live than foods found in their natural state. When it comes to health, who cares about how long a food will last. It is dead food providing your body with no nutrients. This is why nature provides man with plenty of earth so that we can grow plenty of food. When food goes bad, there is another to take its place.

The Process of Refining Foods

A grain of brown rice

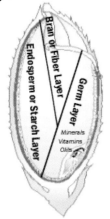

God made

A grain of white rice

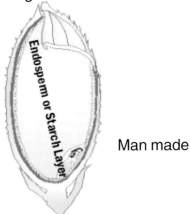

Man made

Brown Rice has a
1) Fiber layer to cleanse out the colon through bowel movements
2) Germ layer to provide the body with nutrients
3) Starch layer drains nutrients from soil but do not contain them

A grain of white rice has
1) Only the starch layer which contains no nutrients, therefore it cannot provide the body with nutrients

Food processing companies now have found a so-called better way to process their breads and cereals. There are enriched breads and cereals, which are supposedly better for us. The processing companies figure that since the public is becoming smarter about their health, they need to come up with a better lie to tell them. Now they are telling us that enriched breads and other enriched foods are healthier for us and they will still have a long shelf life. Enriched foods are better than plain processed foods, but calling enriched foods healthy is not true. When foods are enriched they go through the same bleaching process as plain processed foods, and afterwards, the companies attempt to put a small amount of nutrients that were taken out back into the foods. Why take the nutrients out in the first place? Saying a food is enriched is the same as asking your friend for change for a dollar, and you give him or her a one dollar bill, and he or she only gives you back a nickel. It just doesn't balance out.

When foods are processed, they are totally destroyed, and this is not the way God intended for these foods to be eaten. These processing companies even go as far as to say that these processed foods are natural. When a food is natural, that means that it comes from nature. I have never heard of so many natural foods before. You will not find natural white rice, natural white bread, and natural white sugar. If it does not grow from the earth, then it is not natural, meaning nature does not make it that way. If your diet consists of dead, refined, processed foods, start to eliminate them from your diet today. Begin to eat a majority of God's Original Diet.

Meats

Meats are the most addictive food we can eat. Meals are not complete if they don't include meat. In the early 1900's, only the rich ate meat. Meat was very expensive, and only the rich could afford to eat it. Poor people only ate natural foods, because natural foods were the only foods they could afford and they also grew most of the food they ate. Poor people were pretty healthy in those days. The rich ate high on the hog, cow, and chicken. Unfortunately, only the rich suffered from heart disease, cancer, and artery disease. Poor people did not have such diseases. Unfortunately, today, everyone can afford to eat meat; everyone can afford to eat high on the hog.

When someone asks, "What's for dinner?", they mean, "What meat is being served?." Most commercials on television today are advertising meat. Fast food companies spend millions of dollars advertising that their hamburgers, chicken, or pizza is the best.

Humans will eat almost anything. I have heard of people eating live oysters, monkeys, shark, snakes, alligators, bear, squid, octopus, dogs, cats, and other animals.

Humans have probably eaten every animal alive, just because we are curious about the taste. Humans will eat anything, and some of us have even been known to eat other humans. Enough about those animals, let's talk about the top four animals consumed by humans today - pig, cow, chicken, and fish. These four animals complete almost every meal. These animals are raised for only one purpose - to be eaten. Breakfast, lunch or dinner is not complete if it doesn't include one of these four animals. There is not one holiday that doesn't include one of these four animals. There is not a social event that doesn't include one of these animals.

When excessive amounts of meat are eaten, it is very hard for the body to get rid of it through the GI tract. This is because when the body tries to get rid of breakfast, lunch is coming in. When the body tries to get rid of lunch, dinner is coming in. It takes many hours for our bodies to digest meat. Imagine eating the standard American breakfast of sausage, bacon, and eggs at 8 o'clock in the morning. Then we have the standard American lunch of hamburger, fries, and Coke at 12 o'clock in the afternoon, and at 5 o'clock we have the standard American dinner, which usually consists of chicken or steak and vegetables seasoned in fat back. Our body does not have enough time to digest these heavy meals adequately.

So the body thinks about where it can put the waste. The body usually stores it in the abdomen or lower GI tract, and we become obese. As the meat begins to sit in the lower GI tract for long periods of time, it begins to secrete poisons. These poisons lead to many diseases, such as cancer, arthritis, high cholesterol, heart attack, stroke, high blood pressure, osteoporosis, fibroids, kidney stones, and gallstones.[27,28,29,30,31]

There are many common diseases that could be prevented if only we would decrease our meat intake. We cannot expect to be healthy and full of energy and abuse our bodies by eating these dead foods. I am not telling you to become a vegetarian, but we must start to reduce our excessive meat intake. If you must eat meat, I believe you should eat it no more than three times a week. I feel that red meats such as pork, beef, goat, and lamb should never be eaten. These meats are just too hard for the body to digest and have been linked to many diseases. Eliminate them from your diet if you want to be healthy.

The foods described above are all man-made foods. They have no fiber, no vitamins, minerals, phytochemicals, water, or any other nutrients that your body needs. I am not telling you that you should never eat these foods, but be aware of how these foods affect the body.

> *Proverbs 23:1-3, When thou sittest to eat with a ruler, consider diligently what is before thee: And put a knife to thy throat, if thou be a man given to appetite. Be not desirous of his dainties: for they are deceitful meat*

God's Original Diet   -vs-   **Man-Made Foods**

Healthy Foods cause
1. Stable Weight
2. Reduce Stress
3. Bowel Movements
4. Energy Strength
5. Health
6. Life

Unhealthy Foods cause
1. Obesity
2. Depression
3. Constipation
4. Fatigue
5. Disease
6. Death

If a majority of your diet consists of man-made foods, you may be cursed with sickness leading to an early death, but if a majority of your diet consists of God's Original Diet you will be blessed with abundant life as God intended.

Let's look at how God's Original Diet gives us this abundant life.

V.
WHO SATISFIETH THY MOUTH
WITH GOOD THINGS

Breast Milk

The first food that humans should taste after birth is mother's milk. Sadly, many mothers don't breast-feed, and that starts the path for disease in a child's life. If you don't breast-feed, you are not giving your baby the best. Breast milk is nature's most perfect food for your infant. It is superior to all other milk. Mother's milk provides all the vitamins, minerals, proteins, and nutrients your baby needs. When a mother breast-feeds, more than just milk is given to the child; there are other benefits. Studies have shown that breast-fed babies are smarter than babies raised on other types of milk. Breast-fed babies scored higher on standardized tests and I.Q. exams.[1,2] Breast-fed babies are less likely to be obese because they are not ingesting the growth hormones pumped into cows.[3]

Mothers also benefit from breast-feeding. Breast-feeding creates an emotional bond between the mother and baby. [4] Studies show that mothers who breast-feed are less likely to develop uterine and breast cancer than mothers who do not breast-feed. The studies show that breast-feeding reduces the risk of cancer through structural changes in breast tissue. This is linked with lactation, and it helps the mother's uterus to contract to its normal size and shape more quickly.[5,6] Early breast milk contains colostrum, which contains hormones and antibiotics that help the baby have its first bowel movement with ease and help develop the baby's immune system.[7,8] Breast milk lowers the risk of a baby developing asthma and allergies.[9] Other advantages of mother's milk include it's designed by God especially for babies, it's always at the right temperature, it's easier for babies to digest, and it's free. So breast-feed because it is a win-win for both baby and mother.

All babies are born with an enzyme called lactase. Lactase is the enzyme used to digest milk. After about nine to twelve months of age this enzyme disappears. It just leaves the body for some unknown reason.[10] This is why I believe most people are lactose intolerant after about nine months of age. I believe that this is the body's way of saying it is time for the baby to stop drinking milk and to start eating solid foods.

These foods should be eaten everyday, and they were made by God for us to enjoy and to provide abundant life. After the baby stage, humans were designed by God to eat the following foods.

God's Original Diet

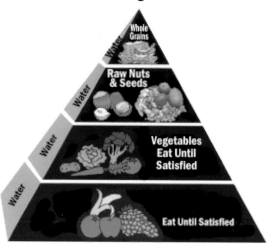

Fruits

> *2 Kings 19:29 And this shall be a sign unto thee, Ye shall eat this year such things as grow of themselves, and in the third year sow ye, and reap, and plant vineyards, and eat the fruits thereof.*

Fruit is probably the healthiest foods to eat. Fruit was the original food given for man to eat. Adam and Eve were fruitarians in the beginning of time, meaning they only ate fruit. Fruit is a cleanser of the body and provides the body with quick energy. Fruits are the easiest of all foods for the body to digest. Our bodies begin to get energy from fruit within minutes after eating it. It takes very little energy from the body to digest fruit, and the body gets a lot of energy in return for digesting it. Fruit provides the body with all the nutrients it needs for survival. Fruit is the best when it comes to cleaning out your GI tract and it only cleans away the toxins and bacteria that the GI tract doesn't need, and leaves the good.

When people hear that they need to start eating fruit ,they make the excuse that fruit doesn't agree with them. This means that fruit makes them have bowel movements. The only reason that you and fruit don't agree is because you are clogged up with toxins and waste, and when you eat fruit it cleanses you out by making you have bowel movements. It is not that fruit does not agree with you; fruit is telling you that you need to be cleaned out. If you have bowel movements every time you eat prunes, raisins, oranges, bananas, or any other fruit, it is the fruit's way of cleaning you out. Fruits are very high in fiber and contain many vitamins, minerals, phytochemicals, fiber, and other nutrients that our body needs in order to survive. Fruits contain no cholesterol, fats, and very little protein. Fruits are very high in carbohydrates, but remember, God's carbohydrates are good for you. Fruits don't clog up arteries, raise blood pressure, or cause obesity. In fact, there has never been a study linking the eating of fruit to heart disease, cancer, strokes, or any disease.

Fruits have a high percentage of sugar that the body needs to survive. The sugar in fruit is converted into glucose, which is the only sugar the brain uses. This sugar provides the body with quick energy. Each fruit has unique nutrients, which makes it different from other fruits.

Melons can make up an entire meal by themselves. Melons should be eaten by themselves, never with any other foods, and always eaten on an empty stomach, preferably when you wake up in the morning. Melons are about 95% water and contain great juices for cleaning the urinary bladder. They are rich in vitamins A, B, and C, and rich in calcium, phosphorus, potassium, and Magnesium. Melons provide a quick source of energy for the body as well.

Oranges are very rich in vitamins A, B, C, and E. They contain about 87% water and plenty of fiber. They are also rich in magnesium, calcium, and potassium. Oranges help fight off many different nutrient deficiency diseases such as scurvy, night blindness, and bone diseases like osteoporosis. They are an acidic fruit, but when they enter the body they have an alkaline effect. It is a great fruit to eat for quick energy and quick cleansing of the GI tract. Oranges also contain carotenoids that fight cancer production in the body.

Apples contain about 85% water and are rich in magnesium, iron, and potassium. They are a good source of vitamins A, B, and C and are good for fighting off fevers and inflammation. Apples are high in fiber and begin to aid the GI tract in digestion within minutes of being eaten. There are many different color variations of apples, ranging from green to yellow. Apples are good for sauces, pies, juices, and salads and are best eaten in their natural raw state.

Bananas contain about 80 to 90% water. Bananas are also rich in potassium, magnesium, and fiber. They also contain vitamins B, and C and are best known for their high carbohydrate content. Many people tell me that they cannot eat bananas because they cause stomach cramps. I find that these people are eating bananas before they're ripe. Bananas should only be eaten when ripe, and they are not ripe until they have brown spots covering the hull. They should never be eaten when green because that means they are not fully matured. The green hull also means that the banana is full of starch, and that the starch has not turned into sugar. This is why people who eat bananas when the hull is green experience stomach cramps, because the starch causes discomfort in the stomach.

Grapes come in many colors and flavors. They are made up of about 80 to 85% water and contain many vitamins, minerals, fiber, and other nutrients the body needs. Grapes should be eaten raw, in their natural state and have been shown to help clean different organs of the body, especially the liver and kidneys. Grapes help eliminate uric acid from the kidneys, which is excessive in arthritis patients. They help fight many illnesses, such as stones in the gallbladder and kidneys. Grapes help clean out the GI tract and prevent many illnesses including obesity.

Lemons and Limes are probably the best cold-fighting food. Like oranges, lemons are acidic but have an alkaline effect in the body. Lemons contain about 90% water and are rich in vitamin C, minerals, phytochemicals, fiber, and other nutrients. Lemon juice has a very strong acid taste, but it is good for fighting colds, the flu, bronchitis, pneumonia, and other mucus-forming illnesses. They can also be used as a natural antiseptic for bruises, cuts, and sores. Limes also have the same qualities as lemons and oranges. Limes are usually sweeter than lemons, but sour compared to the orange. In fact, limes are a product of lemons and oranges. If you have a mucus forming illness such as a cold or flu, these fruits should be used everyday to help fight the illness.

Grapefruit has a sweet and sour flavor. They contain about 90% water and have many vitamins, minerals, fiber, and other nutrients. Grapefruits help prevent diseases such as arthritis and gout by dissolving crystals that are deposited in joints.

Peaches are a good laxative food because of their high fiber content. Peaches contain about 90% water and are rich in vitamins, minerals, and phytochemicals. Peaches help clean both the kidneys and urinary bladder and are also rich in calcium, sodium, and potassium. They are easily digested and have a high alkaline effect on the body.

Pears also act as a good laxative for the body. They contain about 90% water and are rich in vitamins, minerals, and other nutrients.

Pineapples are another citric acid fruit which aids in digestion and helps to fight against kidneys and urinary bladder disease. Pineapples are about 90% water and have a unique taste. They are rich in vitamins B and C, sodium, calcium, and phosphorus. Pineapples also have large amounts of sulphur, chlorine, and potassium, which help aid in digestion and are great cleansers for the body.

Cranberries are one of the few fruits that form an acidic effect in the GI tract and are still beneficial to the body. Cranberries are about 90% water and contain a high amount of natural sulphur. They are also rich in vitamins, minerals, and other nutrients. Cranberries are best known for their cleansing effect on the kidneys and urinary bladder. When eaten raw, cranberries will soften hard stools, making it easier for stools to pass through the bowels. Cranberry juice is also known for softening stones in the kidneys and gallbladder, allowing for better passage through these organs. Cranberries should not be eaten as much as other fruits because of its acidic effect on the body.

Pomegranate fruit is a great food for the intestines. It is rich in vitamins C and E and it has potassium, copper, and iron. It is best known for helping with flatulence (excess gas) and intestinal cramps. It is also helpful in cases of gout and other forms of arthritis.

Avocado is a natural butter and can be used in place of peanut, almond, and other nut butters. It is one of the best sources of fat, containing about 10% fat and 80% water. Avocadoes also provide a good source of natural unsaturated oil. They are rich in vitamins A, B, C, and E and also provide a good source of calcium, magnesium, and phosphorus. Avocados should not be eaten until ripe, when their flesh is soft and tender to the touch. Avocados are great on salads, breads, mixed with vegetables, or just eaten alone.

Olives, like avocadoes, are very rich in unsaturated fat. Olives contain about 14% fat and 75% water. They are also rich in potassium, vitamins, and minerals. Olives should only be eaten when ripe and they are a great source of fat.

Tomatoes are acidic in nature but when eaten have an alkaline reaction in the GI tract. They contain about 97% water and are rich in potassium, calcium, magnesium, and sodium. Tomatoes are also rich in vitamins A, B and C, and they are a great cancer fighting food. Tomatoes should be eaten only when ripe and are good on salads, sandwiches, or eaten alone.

Sugar Cane grows in stalks similar to corn. Chewing cane releases a sweet, tasty juice. It is used for making molasses, which is rich in iron.

Dried fruits should not be eaten as often as fresh fruits, but can be eaten on a regular basis. Try to eat dried fruits that have not been processed or preserved in chemicals. Most dried fruits have been preserved with sulphur or potassium sorbate to improve shelf life and to make the appearance of the fruit more appealing to the buyer. Try to stay away from these processed fruits as much as possible. If dried apricots, raisins, dates, and prunes are orange in color, they have been preserved in sulphur. Dried fruits provide the body with the same nutrients as fresh fruit; the only difference is that the water content has been removed from dried fruits. The fiber is still there and dried fruits are great body cleansers. I think that prunes are the best of all body cleansers. Of course, many people cannot eat prunes because prunes don't agree with them. Dried fruits should be included in your diet, but you should eat more fresh fruits.

If you have not been eating fresh fruit, start today. Eat until full. To be healthy your diet must include fruit. Fruits help to fight off cancers and mucus-forming illnesses such as colds and flu. They help control obesity by keeping the body cleansed, and they help keep toxins out of the body by keeping us regular. Other fruits that can be included in your diet that were not mentioned are: berries (black, goose, straw, rasp and huckleberries), cherries, currants, figs, nectarines, persimmons, plums, strawberries, and papayas. Include as many of these fruits in your diet as possible.

Vegetables

Romans 14:2 For one believeth that he may eat all things: another, who is weak, eateth herbs [vegetables].

Vegetables fall into three classes: 1. leafy greens, 2. flower vegetables , and 3. root vegetables. In the beginning of time, vegetables were not a part of man's diet. In Genesis 1:30 God only gave animals permission to eat vegetables. After Adam and Eve sinned in the Garden of Eden they were driven out and no longer had access to the tree of life, or fruit. God then gave man permission to eat vegetables in Genesis 3:17, 18. **"And unto Adam he said, Because thou hast hearkened unto the voice of thy wife, and hast eaten of the tree, of which I commanded thee, saying, Thou shalt not eat of it; cursed is the ground for thy sake; in sorrow shalt thou eat of it all the days of thy life; 18 Thorns also and thistles shall it bring forth to thee; thou shall eat the herb of the field."** Now man has permission from God to eat vegetables. Vegetables are builders of the body, they build cells and different organ tissues. Fresh vegetables regenerate cells and organ tissues, and provide life and energy to the body. Vegetables provide a good source of proteins, vitamins, minerals, fiber, and other nutrients the body needs to be healthy. Vegetables help fight off many common diseases, and a lack of them in your diet can cause nutrient deficiency diseases.

Broccoli is rich in phosphorus, sulphur, and potassium. It is also rich in vitamin A and B, and folic acid. Broccoli consists of about 90% water and is full of fiber, which helps keep the GI tract clean. It contains sulforaphane, a nutrient that helps to neutralize cancer causing chemicals that damage cells, and it also fights against tumor growth.

Cauliflower is rich in potassium, sulphur, and phosphorus. It is also rich in vitamins, minerals, folic acid, and other nutrients. It is a good cancer fighting vegetable, contains about 90% water, and has a high fiber content.

Asparagus is a tender vegetable made up of about 90% water. Asparagus have a rich supply of sodium, iron, and folic acid and is rich in most vitamins, minerals, and fiber. Asparagus should be eaten raw or slightly steamed because of its tenderness.

Celery contains about 95% water and is rich in organic sodium. It is also rich in vitamins, minerals, and fiber.

Spinach is a green leafy vegetable that consists of about 90% water. It is best known for its rich supply of iron that helps nourish the cells and organ tissues of the body. It is also rich in sodium, calcium, magnesium, as well as fiber and vitamins. Spinach also provides good nutrition for nerves and muscles. Popeye, the sailor man, was the best character to demonstrate how spinach helps nourish muscles.

Carrots are one of nature's most perfect foods. Carrots contain about 90% water and are rich in vitamin A and C. Carrots are also a good source of fiber and contain a rich supply of sulphur, chlorine, and phosphorus. Raw carrots have been shown to be one of a few foods that have all the vitamins, minerals, and nutrients required by the human body, which is why they are one of the most perfect foods we can eat. Carrots probably provide the best source of vitamin A, which is good for night blindness.

Beets are best known for their iron content, which is valuable in nourishing the liver and red blood cells. Beets contain about 90% water and are rich in vitamins, minerals, and other nutrients. Raw beets are effective in relieving constipation and regulating menstrual periods and premature menopause.

Cabbage, both red and white, contains approximately 90% water and is a rich supply of potassium, calcium, and sodium.

Cucumbers contain about 95% water and are rich in iron and magnesium. When fresh, they are very tasty and crispy. They provide a great source of fluorine and silicon, which makes them a great food for growing strong nails, hair, teeth, skin, and bones. Cucumbers should be peeled before eaten, because the hull is very hard for the body to digest.

Lettuce has many varieties, all having nearly the same value to the body. Lettuce contains about 95% water and is a rich source of sodium, calcium, iron, potassium, and magnesium. Lettuce is full of silicon and fluorine, which helps build strong bones, skin, hair, and teeth. Lettuce also helps to soothe ulcers and tumors in the GI tract. Lettuce should always be eaten raw, in salads or alone.

Onions are very rich in carbohydrates and contain about 85% water. They are also rich in potassium, calcium, iron, and silicon. Onions have oils that are very beneficial to the mucus membranes. They have thousands of phytochemicals that help fight against carcinogens and tumors, lowering the risk of colon, stomach, and other cancers. They have been shown to be beneficial to the heart as well. Onions are best eaten raw and are good for seasoning vegetables.

Garlic, like the onion, has many health benefits. Garlic contains about 70% water and is rich in vitamins, minerals, and other nutrients. Garlic is beneficial to the lymph system by helping eliminate toxic waste. Garlic, like the onion, is a valuable cleanser of mucus membranes and is extremely helpful in cleaning the lungs and sinuses in conditions like asthma and colds. Garlic also helps to cleanse the blood, helping conditions like arteriosclerosis and hypertension.

Leeks are part of the onion family and contain about 90% water. Leeks are rich in vitamins B, C and folic acid.

Okra is made up of about 90% water and is valuable in soothing inflamed bowels. Okra also soothes irritations in the urinary bladder, colon, kidneys, and liver.

Potatoes contain about 75% water when raw and are high in carbohydrates. Potatoes are a good source of vitamins A, B, and C. They are good baked, and are best eaten when fresh.

Peppers, usually green, red, or yellow, provide the body with many nutrients. Peppers contain about 90% water and are rich in vitamins. They are also high in fluorine and silicon. Peppers are good on salads, mixed with other vegetables, or just eaten alone. Stay away from hot peppers such as black ground pepper and jalapenos because hot peppers are very irritating to the GI tract, bladder, kidneys, and small intestines.

Peas contain about 75% water when fresh, and are rich in potassium and magnesium.

Sea vegetables, or seaweeds, such as agar-agar, dulse, kelp, kombu, and nori are rich in nutrients. They are rich in vitamins A, B, C, D, niacin, and vitamin B12. Sea vegetables contain a valuable amount of iron, calcium, phosphorus, magnesium, and organic salt. Sea vegetables are great in soups, salads, and eaten with other vegetables.

These are some of the most common vegetables. There are many other vegetables that I did not mention that also provide valuable nutrients to the body. Vegetables should be in our diets everyday.

Vegetables should not be cooked for long periods of time and it is ok to steam them. Try not to season vegetables with meat, salt, sugar, vinegar, or other deadly drugs. If vegetables are not a part of your diet, start including them today. Vegetables help fight against many diseases and help keep our bodies healthy.

> *Psalms 104:14 He causeth the grass to grow for the cattle, and herb for the service of man: that he may bring forth food out of the earth.*

Nuts

Nuts provide the body with valuable amounts of fat and protein. The majority of nuts should be eaten raw because they are full of life. Raw is the way nature provided them for us to eat. Nuts should be eaten in moderation because they are concentrated foods, rich in unsaturated fats and proteins. Mother Nature provides all nuts in shells so that we don't consume them in large amounts.

Almonds contain about 20% protein and are rich in vitamins B, E, iron, calcium, phosphorus, potassium, and magnesium, and are about 50% unsaturated fat. Almonds provide nourishment for bone structure and help strengthen the enamel of the teeth.

Peanuts contain about 25% protein and about 50% of it is made of fat. Peanuts are a good source of vitamins B, E, niacin, iron, and magnesium. Peanuts should only be eaten raw.

Pecans provide a good source of unsaturated fat, making up about 70% of the nut. Pecans consist of about 10% protein and provide the body with a rich supply of nutrients.

Walnuts come in many varieties. The most common three are English, black and white walnuts. Walnuts contain about 20% protein and about 60% unsaturated fat. Walnuts are also rich in vitamin B, E, iron, and zinc.

Brazil nuts are oily, triangular in shape, and very rich in thiamine (vitamin B1), phosphorus, calcium, selenium, copper, and zinc. Brazil nuts are made of about 60% unsaturated fat.

Cashews are bean shaped with a very sweet,unique taste. They are rich in vitamin B, niacin, magnesium, and zinc. Cashews are also a good source of protein, unsaturated fat, and carbohydrates.

Chestnuts are mound-shaped nuts that also have a unique flavor. They are rich in carbohydrates and magnesium and contain about 75% carbohydrates.

Filberts, also called hazel nuts, are rich in unsaturated fat and high in calcium. Filberts contain a rich supply of protein, potassium, magnesium, iron, and vitamins B and C. They are tasty, with a sweet buttery flavor.

Macadamia nuts are grown in Hawaii, Florida and overseas and are usually bought already shelled. They have a sweet buttery taste and are high in fat and low in proteins.

Pignolia nuts, also called pine nuts, also have a sweet buttery flavor. They are high in unsaturated fat and protein. The negative side to pine nuts is that they are very expensive.

Pistachios have a mild flavor and are rich in protein, iron, and potassium. They are usually a pale green color and have a very unique taste.

> *Genesis 2:9 And out of the ground made the Lord God to grow every tree that is pleasant to the sight, and good for food.*

Seeds

Seeds have many nutrients the body needs to fight against many human ailments. Seeds provide a good source of proteins and should be a part of a well balanced diet.

Flax seeds are rich in unsaturated fatty acids and contain a good supply of iron, protein, niacin, phosphorus, and omega 3 fatty acids. Flax seeds help improve the natural glow of hair, skin, and nails. They may also help prevent cancer of the prostate and aid the electrical stability of the heart. Flax seed oils are often used to decrease swelling, sores, and other lesions of the skin. They are used as laxatives to release waste from the bowel. They are great eaten with hot cereals, salads, and breads, or eaten alone.

Sesame seeds are rich in calcium, phosphorus, protein, iron, and unsaturated fatty acids.

Sunflower seeds are rich in protein, vitamins A and B, minerals, and provide a good source of calcium, iron, magnesium, niacin, and potassium. Sunflower seeds contain about 35% protein and about 50% unsaturated fat. Copper, zinc, silicon, and fluorine are also found in sunflower seeds.

Pumpkin seeds contain about 29% protein and are also rich in iron, phosphorus, calcium, zinc, and niacin.

Sprouts seeds are full of enzymes, minerals, and vitamins and provide the body with plenty of energy. Sprouts contain sugars that can be easily digested and used for energy. Sprouts contain vitamins A, B, C, and E, and contain about 90 to 95% water. They are also rich in niacin and folic acid. Some of the most common sprouts are alfalfa, soybeans, peas, butterbeans, lentils, and radish.

Grains

Grains contain about 30 vitamins and minerals and should be a primary source for B vitamins. Grains are also a good source of protein, as well as calcium, magnesium, iron, and phosphorus. Grains are great for breads and cereals. They are full of fiber and help fight off many human ailments. Some common grains are unbleached whole-wheat, flax, brown rice, barley, buckwheat, rye, millet, and oats. Grains should never be eaten processed, refined, or enriched; they should always be eaten as whole grains. Their beneficial nutrients are concentrated in the bran and germ; these both are taken out during processing.

> *Deuteronomy 8:7-8 For the Lord thy God bringeth thee into a good land, a land of brooks of water; A land of wheat, and barley, and vines, and fig trees, and pomegranates; and land of oil olive and honey.*

Fresh Legumes

Legumes, including peas, clovers, lentils, and beans, provide a rich source of protein, vitamins, iron, calcium, phosphorus, and many other nutrients. Fresh legumes are better sources of nutrients than the dried form because the sprouting legumes contain more water than dried legumes. Sprouting legumes also contains more vitamin C than dried legumes and are easier for the body to digest than dried legumes. Fresh legumes contain about 85% water, which makes them similar to fresh vegetables and fresh fruits. Dried legumes have lost their water content, which makes them harder for the body to digest. Dried legumes also have a higher percentage of concentrated protein and carbohydrates. This is why some people have gas after eating dried beans and many other dried legumes.

Dried legumes were designed for cattle, horses, pigs, and other livestock, and should not be eaten by humans. It is important that we eat our legumes fresh, when they are high in water content and nutrients. This makes them easier for the body to digest.[11,12,13,14,15,16]

> *Psalms 34:8 O taste and see that the Lord is good; blessed is the man that trusted in him.*

VI.
The Spiritual Way To Health

What America calls a health care system is really a sick care system. Most people only go to the doctor when they're sick. It is only when we get a severe headache, cold, flu, symptoms of diabetes, cancer, or heart problems that we decide to go to a doctor, and, sadly, most can only offer drugs. Doctors can only treat you if you get sick. If you are healthy, they cannot help you. It is difficult for alternative health physicians to convince patients to be treated while they are healthy so that they remain healthy, but that is true health care.

People have always depended on doctors and other health care providers to give us health. As doctors, we have only made the nation sicker. In countries where there are very few doctors, disease are almost nonexistent. More Americans are taking pills that only cover up symptoms. More Americans are dying from diseases, and, doctors as a whole, still have no clue why. When we get sick and diseased, we put our hopes in doctors, hoping that they will find a miracle pill to fix our disease. As the pharmaceutical companies make more drugs and become rich, we as a nation become sicker. Every time a so-called miracle pill comes on the market, we put our faith in it, and it only lets us down, not living up to its expectations.

Health comes from healthy living. Eating a majority of God's Original Diet helps contribute to maintaining a healthy body, but we should do other things as well. These are things that you have to do in order to be healthy. It's not your doctor's, family's, or spouse's responsibility - it's yours. No one can give you health but God, and it is up to you to keep it. The way you live your life, the way you eat, drink, and the decisions you make in life will eventually determine your health later in life. There are many things that help determine our health, but it is up to us to do them. Yes, diet plays the most important role in determining our health, but we must do other things to be healthy.

Fasting

Isaiah 58:8 After fasting thine health shall spring forth speedily

Fasting is a period of time the body goes without food and drink. During a fasting period, water is the only food you are allowed to drink. A fast can last for hours, days, or months. If foods other than water are consumed or eaten, it is not a fast. It then becomes a diet. There is no such thing as a fruit fast, juice fast, or vegetable fast. There are fruit, juice, and vegetable diets. Only water is consumed during a fast. The reason water is allowed is because water has no nutrients. Water is pure, it is life, and it is a part of the body; after all, the body is made of 75% water. When we drink water, it goes straight through the digestive system and becomes a part of our body. Now, I know this is where I will begin to lose many people. They will think I am crazy. But fasting is mentioned in the Bible many times.

In Isaiah Chapter 58, which is considered the fasting chapter, in verse 8, God promised us that after fasting **"Then shall thy light break forth as the morning, and thine health shall spring forth speedily; and thy righteousness shall go before thee; the glory of the Lord shall be thy reward."** God said many times that man should fast and pray, and I don't think He would ask His people to do anything that would harm us. Fasting is God's way of doing surgery on the body. God asks that His people fast to get closer to Him. Not only should we eat the way God intended for good health, but we should also fast the way God intended for health. Even Jesus, the Son of God, had to fast to get closer to the father, and so should we. Pushing back from food is the hardest thing for man to do. I know preachers who preach and teach the Bible every Sunday who cannot push away from the plate. They read in the Bible that we should fast but just find it hard to do. It is hard to fast because we have learned that we should eat everyday. I remember learning in preschool that you can live only three days without food, so it is important that we eat everyday. It is amazing how the food industry brainwashes kids to believe certain things. They know that if you start them believing as kids, they are brainwashed for life.

Even adults reading this book will not believe what I am saying. Even though it makes sense to you, it is hard to believe this information because you have been brainwashed by man since childhood. We, as humans, love the taste of food and cannot think about what it would be like to be without it, for even short periods of time. Fasting is a way to get close to God because we become humble when we fast. If you need a spiritual answer to any question from God, I guarantee, that if you fast and pray, you will receive that answer. In addition to the great spiritual aspects of fasting, there are many health benefits from fasting.

Please don't ask your doctor about fasting because 99% of doctors don't have a clue about fasting and will discourage you. Who will you believe man or God? Many doctors compare fasting with starvation, which is far from the truth. Fasting is abstaining from foods for a short period of time, with no hunger pains and no major loss of nutrients. Starvation is to suffer or die from a lack of food. Starvation is the time period after fasting where hunger pains are in the stomach and the body starts to lose major nutrients. When people die from lack of food, they die from starvation and not fasting. People can die from starvation, but not from fasting. God would not ask His children to do something that would harm their lives. I feel if a doctor lacks knowledge about fasting, he/she should refer the patient to a doctor that is knowledgeable, and not discourage the patient from fasting.

Often, fasting can be the best thing a person can do for his or her body. Fasting is very important to your health because it gives the body a rest, especially the GI system. Just like your body needs to rest at night, while you sleep, so does your GI tract. Our GI tract does not stop working at night while we sleep because it has to continue working so that our body will have energy and life for the next day.

When we eat everyday, three times a day, and our GI tract never gets a break, it never stops working. Eventually, it will break down with cancers, fatigue, bowel diseases, ulcers, heart disease, and other illnesses. Imagine how you would feel if you continued to work everyday, all day long without ever getting a break and never allowing your body to rest or sleep. Common sense tells us that our bodies would eventually give out and stop because of a lack of energy, right? Our bodies can work for just so long before giving out of energy. This same thing happens with our GI system. When we eat everyday, three or more times a day, our GI system never gets a rest. Keep in mind that most of us are eating heavy, hard-to-digest meats, coffee, sodas, unrefined processed foods, and other deceitful foods. This will only destroy our digestive system because it never stops working. This constant working eventually breaks down the GI tract, which leads to diseases.

Fasting gives the GI tract a rest. Not only does fasting give your GI tract a rest, but it gives the whole body a rest. The heart, kidneys, liver, gallbladder, and other important organs get a much-needed rest. Sure, they still function, but they don't have to work as hard, since there is no food coming into the system. The function of these organs relies on the amount and the type of food coming into the GI system. When our body realizes that we are fasting, it starts to get rid of toxins and waste that we have put in our bodies over the years. This is when we experience headaches, diarrhea, dizziness, vomiting, sweating, nausea, and other symptoms because this is the body's way of getting rid of the toxins.

Many times when we experience these symptoms, we become frightened and go back to eating again, and the symptoms go away. In reality, this is the body's way of telling us that we need to fast and starts to clean us out, because when we stop eating, our body focuses energy on getting rid of toxins. The body says, "Since there is no food coming in, now I have time to get rid of all the waste inside me." But as soon as we start to eat again, the body has to focus its energy back on digesting the food, and the symptoms go away. It is important to know the symptoms you will experience from fasting before you begin.

When you fast and experience these symptoms, don't become frightened. Try to tolerate the discomfort for a short period of time, and you will experience great energy and health in the end. People who already eat healthy foods don't experience these symptoms when they fast. I have never said that fasting is easy, but with God, and a made-up mind, all things are possible. All good things are worth making a sacrifice for, and your health is worth fasting for. The nature of one's illness determines the length of time a person should fast. When experiencing the symptoms of fasting, we just have to bear with the symptoms until our body is cleansed. After the symptoms are gone, we will feel much better, have more energy, and will be glad that we were able to defeat the symptoms.

At least two days before fasting, we should eat only fruits and vegetables. It is also important that we drink plenty of water when we fast because water goes through the body, especially the liver and kidneys, and flushes out toxins that have accumulated in the body from years of eating deceitful foods. Pure distilled water is preferred. When we come off a fast and return to eating food, it is important that we break the fast with easy to digest foods because our GI tract is rested. The GI tract contracts or shortens when we fast, which means we need to feed it foods that are easy to digest so that the GI tract will start to digest food properly.

Fruits, vegetables, and their juices are the foods of choice to break a fast because they are the easiest to digest and provide the quickest energy. Also, their fiber will help continue to cleanse the body. If we break our fast by eating unhealthy foods, it causes our stomach to cramp, and we experience much pain in the bowels because our body is not ready to start digesting heavy foods immediately after a fast. Therefore, it is important to eat healthy foods before and after a fast.

When an illness is resolved by fasting, it is important that we continue to eat healthy after the fast so that we will not be prone to develop the illness again. If we continue to eat unhealthy food after a fast, it defeats the purpose of fasting in the first place. Let's take a look at a person with high blood pressure, for example. The reason a person has high blood pressure is usually because they eat heavy, fatty meats which clog the arteries, season every food with salt, live stressful lives, drink coffee, sodas, teas, and eat other unhealthy foods. If the person fasts for a few days (usually 3 to 10 days) the heart gets a rest, the body cleans out the arteries, and the blood pressure usually falls.

After the fast, if the person eats healthy live foods his blood pressure will remain normal, but if he goes back to eating heavy meats, salt, coffee, and keeps stress in his life, his blood pressure will rise again. It is very important that we continue to eat healthy foods after fasting.

How do we know when we need to fast? There are many ways the body tells us that we need to fast, but humans, as a whole, don't understand or listen to the signs. When you are sick with colds, flu, bronchitis, high blood pressure, diabetes, etc., and many other illnesses, it is our body's way of telling us we need to fast.

Let's take a look at colds, for example. Have you ever noticed that when you have a cold you normally don't have an appetite? This is your body's way of telling you not to eat, so that it can focus its energy on getting rid of mucus and other toxins. Instead, many of you eat a meal or take medicine, and your body then has to focus its energy on digesting the meal or getting rid of the medicine. Since you don't have an appetite when you get a cold, it is important not to eat until you've gotten over the cold. Your appetite will come back when the cold is gone.

Even animals know the importance of fasting. If a dog in the wild gets sick, it will fast. You can put all the food you want to in its face and it will not eat. Dogs will continue to fast while they are sick. After the sickness has resolved, they will start to eat grass, a natural food that provides medicine for them. There are many animals that fast when they are sick - bears, snakes, dogs, and cats. We, as humans, can learn a lot from animals. Many spiritual leaders fast, and many religions allow their members to fast periodically. In the Bible Moses, David, Elijah and Jesus fasted for forty days. Now I am not asking you to fast that long, but these are great Biblical examples we can learn from.

Fasting is a great way to cleanse out the body, and people have had great results with it. Some benefits of fasting are that it is the safest way to lose weight, it gives the whole body a well-deserved rest, it cleanses your bloodstream, and it breaks down plaque built up in the arteries from years of eating fatty foods. It gives the heart a rest so it decreases your blood pressure, and it decreases tumor growth. Diseases that have great results from fasting are obesity, asthma, allergies, high blood pressure, high blood cholesterol, arthritis, diabetes, uterine fibroids and other tumors, impotence, poor eyesight, early stages of cancer, heart disease, atherosclerosis, kidney and liver disease, GI tract diseases, prostate tumors, tuberculosis, and a host of other illnesses.[1,2,3]

I grew up with a fasting mother. My mother has fasted forty days and nights many times, and I have never seen her suffer from any major sickness. My mother may have had a common cold twice, that I can recall, because she allows her body to be cleansed through fasting. My mother fasted for spiritual reasons, but at the same time she was cleansing her physical body. Now, I realize that fasting is not only a way to get close to God, but a way to get healthy as well.

Fasting has many benefits, but temptations come along with it. Every time you decide to fast, for spiritual or physical reasons, a temptation will appear from out of the blue. Whether it be friends or family tempting you with food, watching food commercials on television, or someone telling you that you are crazy to fast (because they are ignorant), you can always count on something strange happening before or during a fast. For example, I was fasting one day, and a man who I did not know came out of nowhere and handed me a watermelon. He told me, "I know that I don't know you, but I want you to have this." Now that's strange. Many times when my mother would fast, neighbors would bring her cakes and pies and other foods. It is odd how these things happen when you are fasting. Well, if Jesus was tempted to turn stone into bread when he was fasting (St. Matthew Chapter 4), then we do not stand a chance of avoiding temptation when we fast. So if you decide to fast, don't be surprised if someone tempts you to do or eat something you don't want to. Often the tempter is someone close to you.

If you are interested in fasting, consult a doctor who is trained in fasting before you begin a fast. Remember, God told his people to fast, and we should trust him before any man.

> *Joel 2:12 Therefore saith the Lord, turn ye to me with all your heart, and with fasting.*

Exercise

> *Psalms 104:5 Who satisfieth thy mouth with good things; so that thy youth is renewed like the eagle's.*

Exercise plays an important role in staying healthy. Exercise should be a part of our lives everyday, in some form or another. It would be nice if we could just lie around and watch television, drink Kool-aid, and eat ice cream all day, and still be healthy. Unfortunately, staying healthy isn't that easy. Exercise plays a major role in the development of our muscles; and without exercise, our muscles cannot perform their job of moving the body. If muscles are not exercised they lose their function. There is an old saying, "If you don't use it, you lose it." And this is true. If we don't use our muscles, then we lose them, usually to fat. That is when we turn to weight loss pills and diets.

You can always find gimmicks and pills that claim that if you use them, you don't have to exercise. There are even pills on the market that are supposed to exercise for you, while you rest or watch television. Exercise in a bottle. In order to be healthy, we have to get off our sorry behinds and get active. If you are waiting for a pill to lose weight for you, you may lose your life instead. Ever since the invention of the automobile, television, fast food, weight loss pills, and vitamins, Americans have exercised less. Even though some of these inventions are good, they should not take the place of exercise. These inventions have made us, as a nation, very lazy. Before these inventions came along, obesity was not as prevalent as it is today.

There are many healthy benefits to exercise. Exercise helps build up your immune system and it allows you to get rid of toxins through sweating and breathing. It may help prevent premature aging and provide good skin tone. [4] Exercise helps the bowels flow properly, and it helps to normalize blood pressure. Studies show that exercise helps prevent, control, and even reverse diabetes, obesity, cancer, arthritis, and many other diseases. [5, 6, 7, 8] Exercise helps to strengthen every muscle in the body.

There is one muscle that must be exercised on a regular basis because it is very important to the survival of the body. The most important muscle in the body is the heart, a muscle about the size of your fist that is protected by the rib cage. This muscle pumps blood to every other muscle, therefore it is important that we keep the heart healthy. When the heart is healthy, the rest of the body is healthy; but when the heart is sick, the rest of the body is sick. By keeping the heart healthy through exercise you can prevent, control, and even reverse many heart diseases.[9] The best way to exercise the heart is through walking. Walking is the best exercise for your body. Almost every muscle functions when we walk. Sometimes our heart needs to be stimulated, and brisk walking and running will do that. Running helps to speed up our heart rate and gives it a good workout. It doesn't make sense to workout your arm and leg muscles and never workout your heart by walking or running.

We should exercise the heart at least three times a week with brisk walking or running. Running promotes osteoblastic formation of bone. That means that when you run, old bone is being replaced by new bone. This helps reduce our chance of having bone diseases like osteoporosis. [10] When we are inactive, old bone is never replaced by new bone, it is replaced by fat. Have you noticed that people who don't exercise often have swollen legs and ankles - especially obese people? When you don't exercise, your body doesn't circulate enough blood through the organs that help eliminate toxins from the body. Due to gravity and lack of exercise, toxins settle in the feet and ankles and cause swelling. As soon as these people start to exercise, the swelling goes down.

It is important to exercise for 30 minutes at least 2 to 3 times a week to keep our bodies in good shape. If you are not exercising for health reasons, ask your doctor about an exercise program that is appropriate for you. There are many forms of exercise that have beneficial results, but remember, to keep that heart muscle exercised. If your heart doesn't pump blood to other muscles properly, the purpose of exercise is defeated. Exercises that are helpful to the body are stretching, walking, running, swimming, weightlifting, football, basketball, and any form of exercise that speeds up the heart rate. Our bodies are designed for movement and activity, not to sit around all day and be inactive. The body is made up of over 200 bones and over 640 muscles. All the physical motions of the body involve muscle activity, whether it is the heart beating, skeletal movements, bowel movements, eating or sexual activity; it takes muscles to perform physical motions. If we don't keep our bones and muscles active, the result is obesity, sickness, and disease. It is important that your body stay active because, remember, if you don't use your body you will lose your body.

Rest and Sleep

Genesis 49:15 And he saw that rest was good.

Rest and sleep are very important for good health. Rest is a period of time during which the body is inactivite so that it can restore or recharge energy lost during the day. It is estimated humans spend about one-third of their lives sleeping. It is important to reward our bodies with quality rest. Experts believe that the average person should sleep at least eight hours a night. From a common sense point of view, you should rest when tired, and your body will awaken when it has gotten the proper amount of sleep. This may take eight, ten, twelve, or even more hours.

The best sleep occurs during the hours before midnight, due to lack of sunlight. It is harder for the body to rest during the day because of sunlight. Sunrays stimulate the pituitary gland, making the body think it should be awake, and not asleep. But due to a variety of work schedules, people have to sleep when they can. It was originally planned that man would work during the day and rest at night, but everyone can't do that. Rest provides a way for the body to repair and rejuvenate itself with energy and relaxes and refreshes muscles, nerves, and the brain. Rest contributes to peace of mind, body, and spirit. When you rest there should be no worries, stress, and distractions. Sleep gives the eyes a rest at night so that you can have good vision the following day.[11]

Unfortunately, there are many people in our society who don't get the proper amount of rest their bodies deserves. Many people have so much drama and stress in their lives that they don't have time to rest. We get so much in debt that we can't afford not to work. We have bad marriages and divorces stressing us out, causing us to lose sleep. Eating unhealthy foods can also have an affect on the quality of sleep and rest. When drama comes into our lives, and we can't sleep, we start to take drugs. Drugs don't give the body good rest because they affect the nervous system.

In order to sleep the nervous system has to relax and it is hard for the body to relax when it's full of toxins. When stress is in the body, your muscles contract and become tight which can cause headaches that will keep you from relaxing.

Stress is probably the biggest reason that many people don't get enough sleep and rest. It is important that we keep our stress to a minimum. I know that there are many stresses that we cannot control, but we have to eliminate bad stress from our lives. Stress is not worth losing good quality sleep over because it will eventually cause you to make bad decisions in life. If you are not getting satisfying, peaceful, and healthy rest at night or during the day, start to eliminate the things that may be causing you stress. Start to earn your rest by doing physical activities. Go for a walk or run in the evening. Walk the dog or swim in the pool. Play basketball or other physical sports. Rest is something that should be earned with both physical and mental activity. You will never see any other animal taking pills in order to sleep. Only human lives become so fast paced that we need pills to put us to sleep. Other animals in the wild play and stay active, and sleep and rest comes naturally to them. You will find that when you start to become active you will not need a pill to help you relax and fall asleep. Your rest and sleep will come naturally, and it will be a satisfying, peaceful rest.

Reduce Stress

Stress is a part of life that we cannot avoid. It is something that we just have to learn to live with. Stress does play an important role in our lives, but the way we react to stress is even more important. It is important to not let stress control us; we must control it. We should learn to always stay calm and cool under pressure so we can make good decisions. Stress causes many people to make the wrong decisions in life. We are stressed by traffic in the morning on our way to work, we have financial stresses, stressful relationships with family, co-workers, significant others, and many other stressful events.

We must learn to manage stress, which will allow us to make good decisions. Stress is tension, which affects our bodies and our minds, impacting our attitudes, behavior, and decisions. Stress is caused by our reaction to life's changes. Our bodies and minds react to stress, seeking to maintain equilibrium or balance in our lives. The tension of stress is felt in different regions of the body, causing muscles to tighten or contract. These contractions will cause headaches, backaches, stomachaches, and other illnesses of the body. Even though there are no studies on this, I feel that stress is the number one killer in America. Many diseases that Americans suffer from can all be related to stress. Asthma, diabetes, ulcers, heart attack, and stroke have all been linked to stress [12]. I feel that depression, anxiety, hypochondria, schizophrenia, and many other psychological illnesses are all related to stress as well.

Stress is a part of life and it is impossible to live without it. People have different reactions to stress because we are all different. What may make me angry may not even affect another, and vice versa. There are many physical and mental reactions to stress which include anxiety, anger, increased muscle tension, rapid shallow breathing, and an increase in blood pressure, blood sugar, and heart rate. These reactions affect every system in the body, especially the nervous, endocrine, immune, and GI systems. Stress affects how well the body digests food and affects how well the body protects you from invading viruses and bacteria.[13] Stress can be good or bad for the body.

There are many ways to manage stress. Stretching and exercising tend to be very helpful with stress, because these two activities cause the body to release toxins. Exercise increases the body's ability to use more oxygen, which causes efficient lung and heart function, which increases the blood supply to muscles. This allows a person to cope with stress for longer periods of time without exhausting the muscles. Relaxing helps with stress, taking pressure off the muscles and bones.

While relaxing, take deep breaths; your body will relax better. Prayer and meditation are effective ways of dealing with stress and should be practiced daily to help control our lives. Taking time out to gather thoughts and focus on our blessings will also help reduce stress. Helping others tends to relieve stress. There is no better feeling than knowing that you have helped someone. Talking also helps to take stress off the body. When we keep feelings inside and don't express them to others, we become depressed, sick, and eventually become stressed out. Talk to someone who you can share your problems with, such as a pastor, family member or doctor. Women are great at talking and sharing their feelings. This may be a reason they live longer than men because men tend to keep things inside without expressing them.

A massage is a great way to help reduce stress. Massaging the muscles causes them to relax, thus releasing tension. Probably the greatest stress releaser is the chiropractic adjustment. Stress can cause bones in the spine to subluxate, which means two bones are misaligned, but the joint surfaces remain intact. Activities of daily living such as walking, running, sitting in front of a computer all day, and even eating unhealthy foods, can cause stress on the body. The body has to put the stress somewhere, so it puts the stress on the spine, causing the body to be subluxated in different areas of the spine. The body tends to place stress in the lower back, buttocks, the lower neck, and upper back. Stress can cause these joints of the spine to become fixated, or not moveable. The chiropractic adjustment is a controlled force to the spine, which puts the vertebra, bones of the spine, back in their proper place, thereby causing the spine to become more moveable. This causes the muscles connected to the bones of the spine to relax, relieving the stress.

Unhealthy foods can put a lot of stress on the body because it takes longer for the body to digest them, and the body usually gets no energy in return for digesting them. Unhealthy foods put stress on every organ in the body. It takes many hours for the body to digest meats, putting unnecessary stress on the body. It takes one day for the kidneys to filter sodas, coffee, and tea, causing them much stress. Many man-made foods lead to sickness and disease that our bodies try to fight off, which is very stressful. This is why our country is overwhelmed with different diseases. Start eating healthy foods that grow from the earth and stop putting stress on your body. Give your body the nutrients and the health it deserves. Eat a diet full of fruits, vegetables, nuts, seeds, and whole grains. These foods put less stress on the body's digestive process. As you begin to eat more of these foods, you will see that you are able to handle stress better.

Pure Air

There is no such thing as pure air anymore. Since the invention of planes and cars and other forms of transportation, pure air is a thing of the past. Farmers spray herbicides, insecticides, and pesticides which pollutes the air. There is no such thing as clean air for people growing up in big cities like Los Angeles, Atlanta, and New York. These cities are trying to get their residents to take local trains and busses to work and social events to reduce pollution. Car-pooling is also an option. On sunny days in many cities you can almost cut the air with a knife, and you can hardly breathe. People who suffer from allergies and asthma are advised to not even come outside on some days, and those who have healthy lungs have a great chance of their lungs becoming infected. We must start to take care of the air we now have; it may not be pure, but it is all we have.

There are a couple of ways that Mother Nature tries to clean the air. Rain cleans the air by washing away toxins. Air smells much cleaner and fresher after a good rain. Trees and other plants convert carbon dioxide, the waste of humans, into life-giving oxygen. Air is essential for our lives. It purifies the body and it energizes the cells in the body. Without air, of course, we would die. The human body can live months without food, but can only survive about 10 minutes without air. Breathing allows air to enter the body and get rid of toxins. Breathing also allows us to receive oxygen from the air which is carried by the blood into the lungs. Oxygen purifies the blood and cells in the body on a regular basis so that it can function properly. If cells and blood don't get purified with oxygen regularly, we die. Oxygen is carried by the blood into the lungs where it is exchanged for carbon dioxide. Carbon dioxide (CO_2) is a deadly chemical formed inside the body and is released from the body when we exhale. When we inhale we breathe in life giving oxygen, and when we exhale we release deadly toxins. Our bodies are constantly creating toxic chemicals that need to be released.

Breathing is just one way these toxins are released. Exercise, bowel movements, perspiration, and urination are other ways we release carbon dioxide and other toxins. If we don't get enough oxygen in our bodies when we breathe, then we don't release enough carbon dioxide either. When life-giving oxygen is not coming in, and toxins are not going out, they accumulate in the body which can cause many respiratory diseases like lung cancer and emphysema. The body cannot get oxygen with these diseases. Not only does this prove that we should breathe in pure air, but we should breathe deeply. Clean air has more oxygen, and the deeper we breathe the more oxygen enters the body. When we breathe deeply, our breaths are longer, which causes the respiratory system to work less. Animals that breathe long and deep breaths usually live longer than those that don't. Rabbits, mice, dogs, and other fast-breathing animals have shorter lives than animals that breathe slower, such as cows and horses.

One of the best ways to get a good quality of air flow is by walking and running. When we run, the body's demand for oxygen is increased, thereby releasing more C02 from the body.

Open up windows to allow fresh air to come into your home. Even when you sleep, crack the window to allow fresh air to enter. Remember, when we exhale we are breathing out C02 which is toxic to our bodies. If we are in a closed tight room where no oxygen can enter, it is possible for C02 to build up and cause sickness in the body. If we breathe in fresh air while we sleep, we wake up feeling refreshed. But if we sleep with our windows closed air-tight, we can wake feeling irritable and cranky because we are full of toxins. Allow fresh air to enter your lungs while you sleep. If it is cold outside, slightly crack the window, just enough to allow fresh air to enter. Just like you need to crack windows in a car to keep carbon monoxide from poisoning the body, we should also crack windows in the home to keep C02 from poisoning the body. Try to practice deep breathing for 5 to 10 minutes when you wake up in the morning, and before you go to bed at night. Deep breathing is the best way to allow good quantity of air to flow into the body and release toxins.

It is important that we plant trees for oxygen. Trees and other plants are our only supply of oxygen in the air. When we cut them down to build houses, cities, unnecessary roadways, and farm land, we are loosing our supply of oxygen. There are many rainforests that are being destroyed because of man's stupidity.

For every tree we cut down, we should plant a tree to take its place. Trees and animals both need each other for survival. Trees and animals live off each other's waste products - oxygen is the waste product of trees, and carbon dioxide is the waste product of humans. Trees need carbon dioxide to survive, and humans and animals need oxygen to survive. Trees use our waste product, carbon dioxide, and turn it into oxygen. Humans and other animals use oxygen, the waste product from trees, and turn it into carbon dioxide. It is amazing how the Creator made us to be of help to each other.

Hardly any trees grow in cities with smog problems, where you can hardly breathe. These cities are full of houses, cars, and plenty of highways with no trees in sight to turn carbon dioxide into oxygen. Trees provide our cities with clean air for us to breathe. Cities with lots of trees are able to use the waste of cars and animals, and turn it into oxygen. The cleanest and freshest air will be found as far away from the city as possible. Country air is the freshest air because there is less traffic, and, therefore, fewer toxins in the air. The country usually has more trees than the city so the trees in the country can use all the carbon dioxide given off by humans and convert it into oxygen. There is also less stress in the country, mainly because there is less to do, meaning less trouble to get into. Have you noticed that country people live longer than city people? This is because country people have less stress, fewer worries, cleaner air, and they grow most of the food that they eat. The country is full of trees and provides the best quality of air to breathe. The cleaner the air, the better your health.

Water

> *Daniel 1:12 And let them give us water to drink.*

Water is the best essential food we can feed our body. Water, along with air, is critical to our bodies. Water is involved in every bodily function, and it is essential for life. All living things need water for their survival; without water, plants, and animals die. Without water, no plant can germinate and grow, and no life would exist. Water provides life to every living thing, therefore water is life. The human body is made up of about 70% water; therefore it is critical that we provide it with a good supply of water. The planet earth is about 70% water also. The same minerals and nutrients that are found in the human body are also found in earth. Most fruits and vegetables are between 70 to 90% water. It is ironic that everything that needs water for survival is made up of about the same percentage of water that the earth has. Plants need the earth's nutrients to grow, humans and animals need plants to survive, and Mother Nature needs humans to take care of her. The best water to drink is pure distilled water. Just like air, there is no such thing as pure water today. Man has polluted the waters with human and animal waste, oils, chemicals, pesticides, and other pollutants. [14]

These pollutants kill the fish, birds, seals, and other animals that live in water. The waste of cattle, pigs, chickens, and other animals raised for their meat pollute our waters.[15] Man has added many harmful chemicals to our drinking water. Chemicals such as chlorine, fluorine, and other harmful chemicals are added to water for treatment and pollute the water even more. Chlorine is a chemical with an irritating gas used as laundry bleach. Would you drink bleach? Probably not. Studies have shown that there may be a link between consumption of chlorinated drinking water and an increased risk for rectal, bladder, and even brain cancer.[16,17,18]

Fluorine is another deadly man-made poison added to drinking water. Fluorine is a toxic, flammable, and irritating gas used in rat and roach poisons. It is also used as a pesticide. High levels of fluorine cause the mottling of teeth and loss of bone density (cavities). Fluorine is found in toothpaste, and dentists and other doctors are telling you that it is good for your teeth. They are telling you that it helps to fight against cavities when, in fact, if used in excessive amounts, it causes cavities.[19]

The animal industry alone produces about 50% of all the water pollution in the United States, in addition to pesticides, herbicides, insecticides, and toxic waste that are put in our waters.[20] When man pollutes the waters, he pollutes the human body at the same time. When our waters become diseased so do our bodies. National Cancer Institute statistics show that the incidence of many cancers, including urinary, testicular, breast, and others, may be linked to drinking contaminated water.[21]

There is nothing in the body that does not consist of water. Every organ, gland, bone, or structure in the body is made up of mostly water. The brain is about 80% water, the lungs are 80% water, blood is 90% water, muscles are 75% water , and even your teeth are made of about 10% water. All structures in the body are made of water, and without it we could not function. Water is used to carry nutrients to various parts of the body for survival. Water is needed to carry out the functions of the heart, liver, kidneys, and other organs for digestion, elimination, for metabolism, and energy. Water helps to get rid of toxins in our body and plays an important role in getting rid of waste through the intestines. Every function in the body that helps to get rid of waste relies on water. Sweating, breathing, bowel movements, and urination all rely on water. Water allows us to bend our joints without friction. Water allows us to bend and flex our bodies without organs touching each other. Water helps to keep our joints lubricated which can prevent arthritis and joint pain. Water helps to protect our arteries, veins, capillaries, and other blood vessels from diseases such as arteriosclerosis. Water helps to keep you looking younger and slows down the aging process. Water helps to relieve stress, which can help prevent sickness and disease.

As you can see, there are practically no bodily functions that occur without water. It helps keep the body at a normal temperature. When our body temperature gets over heated, we sweat to cool off. When our body gets cold, we shiver to bring in heat to the body. Water plays a vital role in the chemistry of life. Water also helps to relieve stress. There is nothing more relaxing than listening to the water at a waterfall, or taking a warm bath. Water helps to relax muscles. Have you noticed how relaxing it is at the beach? Just being around water relaxes the body.

When you drink pure distilled water you are drinking water in its purest form, and that's what the body deserves. You should never drink polluted water in any form. Don't be fooled by companies that sell bottled water. The standards required by state and federal governments for bottled water are the same as standards for tap water.

That's right, bottled water must meet the same standards as the water that comes out of your faucet. Water that you thought was coming from a spring or a clean water source may be coming from someone's faucet.[22] This means that the real source of bottled water may not be known and bottling companies can lie to the public legally, telling them that their water comes from a spring. The Environmental Protection Agency (EPA) has proposed that bottled and drinking water may contain no more than approximately 90 chemicals and other contaminants.[23]

Water should make up the majority of your liquid intake. It is o.k. to drink freshly squeezed fruit and vegetable drinks a couple of times a week, but the majority of your liquid intake should be water. Other animals in nature only drink water. You will never see any animal in nature drinking sodas, Kool-aid, teas, alcohol, or even freshly squeezed fruit drinks. They drink water, and only water, and don't suffer from diseases like man.

People often ask when and how much water they should drink. There have been many answers to this question, but let's use a common sense approach. We should drink water when we get thirsty, and stop drinking it when we are full. Now, I know that might sound a little crazy, but it works. This might sound a little different from the answers you have heard before. I see people carrying bottled water with them everywhere they go. They drink a bottle of water almost every five minutes, because they have heard some so-called health expert say drink plenty of water.

I know experts say to drink 8 to 10 glasses of water a day, and there may be good reason to do that. If one person needs 10 glasses of water a day, it does not mean the next person will need 10 glasses. Just because a 250 pound man needs to drink 12 glasses of water a day does not mean that a 100 pound female needs to drink the same amount. People have their own unique makeup, and what will satisfy one person may not satisfy another. This is known as Biochemical Individuality. Let's learn to listen to our bodies. Your body will let you know when it needs water to drink, because you will become thirsty. It is the proper way the body communicates. Your body will let you know when to stop drinking by giving you a feeling of being full and satisfied. So drink when you get thirsty, and stop drinking when you are full.

If we eat dead foods that don't have any water in them we get thirsty and desire more water to drink. People who eat unhealthy dead foods should drink more water than people who eat healthy foods. People who are on unhealthy diets also get thirsty at a faster rate than people who eat healthy foods because dead foods contain no water. The body becomes thirsty because it needs extra water to digest the dead meals. Of course, if we are eating unhealthy foods, we probably try to quench our thirst by drinking sodas, Kool-aid, and other toxic liquids. Water is the only drink that can satisfy thirst. When you drink coffee, sodas, and other pollutants, they make you even thirstier because the salts and other toxic chemicals in them draw valuable water out of the cells in order to get rid of the chemicals. If we eat life-giving foods that grow from the earth, we don't get thirsty as fast because these foods already contain water. When we eat a healthy diet, we don't have to worry about how much water to drink because we get a great supply from the foods we eat. Do not drink water while eating. Water should be drunken 30 minutes before eating and 1 hour after eating. Water does not need to be digested because it is a part of us. It is readily absorbed through the stomach into the bloodstream, ready for its functions. Start to add more life to your health today by drinking more distilled water and eating foods that grow from the earth.

Sunlight

Genesis 1:16-18 And God made two great lights; the greater light to rule the day: and God saw that it was good.

The sun has always been a controversial issue when it comes to health. There is always some so-called health expert telling us that too much sun can cause cancer. Other experts advise that humans should not get any sunlight. Television commercials tell people to use sun-tanning lotion during the summer, to protect us from the sun's harmful rays. We are told that the sun causes cancer, as if the sun serves no other purpose. We are told that the sun is bad for the skin and eyes, and that we should stay out of the sun as much as we can. Let's think about that and use a common sense approach. Who made the sun? God. Do you think God would make something that would give His people cancer and cause any other harm? No. Well, we should not believe all these lies about the sun.

When God made the sun, he saw that it was good, not that it would give you cancer. The reason that so many people get skin cancer is not because of the sun, it is because of the way man is destroying the planet. Remember, Mother Nature always wins in the end. Other animals in nature spend most of their lives in the sun, and they never have cancers. The sun shines on the food we eat, and it never destroys the food. So why does the sun give humans cancer? Let me explain. The sun has a natural covering called the ozone layer which protects us from its rays. About 50 years ago we hardly heard of people getting skin cancer, but lately it has been on the rise, and the sun is to blame. Ever since the invention of cars, planes, trains, buses, and other forms of transportation, we have polluted the air tremendously.

Fluorocarbons found in cooking sprays, paint spray cans, and air-conditioning help pollute the air as well. Coal factories and factories that produce excessive smoke and toxins also help pollute the air. These chemicals and toxins from different sources rise in the air and cause chemical reactions with the ozone layer, destroying what is supposed to protect the earth from the sun's harmful rays.[24] This is why we hear experts say that there is a hole in the ozone layer. As we continue to pollute the air, these toxins continue to eat through the ozone layer, and the hole continues to get wider. The wider the hole in the ozone becomes, the less protection we have to block the sun's rays. This, along with the fact that their bodies are full of toxins from the food they eat and lifestyle they live, is why more and more people are getting skin cancer.

Skin cancer is caused by eating excessive amounts of fatty foods, smoking, drinking, and living an unhealthy lifestyle. As we eat these foods, they begin to form poisons and toxins in our body, which are absorbed in the skin, colon, breast, prostate, kidneys, and every other organ in the body. When these toxins in the skin are exposed to sunlight for long periods of time, cancer begins to form; it is like cooking meat and fatty foods all over again in the body. You don't see people who eat a majority of God's Original Diet with skin cancer. Animals in the wild spend much of their afternoons in the sun and they never get skin or any other type of cancer. So skin cancer has nothing to do with the sun, it is because man continues to pollute the earth and his body that we must reap the effects of skin cancer and other diseases.

Now that we know that it is man's fault that the sun may cause cancer, let's talk about the benefits of the sun. Without the sun there would be no life. We all know that the sun provides us with light by day, but you may not know that the sun plays a very important role in good health. The sun provides the body with solar energy. Every living creature on this planet has to use solar energy from the sun in order to live. Whether it is fruits, vegetables, animals of any kind, insects or rodents, they all need the sun to survive. The sun gives us both light and health, and, if it were not for the sun, there would be no life. So who cares about cancer, the benefits of the sun greatly outweigh the risks. There are many diseases that come from the body not getting enough sunlight. All animals, including humans, need the sun's rays on their bodies.

The sun gives solar energy to the muscles, nerves, glands, and other organs of the body to help them function properly. The sun has been helpful in nervous problems such as anxiety, and it helps to relieve stress. Sunshine causes the nerves and muscles to relax because the nerves begin to absorb the rays of the sun, and use it for energy.

Sunlight helps lower blood pressure, blood cholesterol, and high sugar levels.[25,26] It helps you sleep and breathe easier. Sunlight is even beneficial to patients with multiple sclerosis.[27]

To prove that the sun is needed for life, we can use green grass as an example. Healthy grass is green and full of life. As long as grass has exposure to sunlight it will remain green. If you put a piece of wood, bricks or any type of covering over grass for a period of about two days, the grass underneath the covering will start to turn yellow and brown. This is because the coverings are blocking the sun's rays from reaching the grass. If the grass stays covered for long periods of time, it will wither and die, because it is starving for sunlight. If you uncover the grass and expose the grass to sunlight again, it will come back to life. The same happens with our bodies.

It is important to expose our bodies to the sun's life-giving rays. People with pale skin are starving for the rays of the sun to provide their body with a healthy glow. Of course, we should not stay in the sun for long periods of time because of the way man has destroyed the ozone layer, but it is vital to our health that we expose our bodies to the sun. The best time to use the sun for solar energy is the early morning or the late afternoon. The sun's rays are not as hot during these times. All animals in nature take advantage of the sun's life giving rays. Lions, tigers, crocodiles, dogs, cats, cows, horses, and other animals in the wild love to lie in the sun and absorb its life giving solar rays, and they never get skin cancer. So what makes humans any different?

The sun also helps grow the foods that we should eat from the earth. This means that each time we eat foods that grow from the earth we are eating foods that have life giving solar energy in them, meaning they also provide your body with solar energy. Sunlight also provides plants with chlorophyll - the blood of the plant. Chlorophyll contains all the nutrients found in plants. When fruits and vegetables grow from the earth, they absorb solar energy from the sun. When we eat these foods, our bodies use the solar energy in the food and turn it into human energy. It is essential that we give our bodies life-giving plant foods that grow from the earth.

Sunlight stimulates the production of vitamin D when it is exposed to the skin. Sunlight is the best source of vitamin D, which is essential for normal bone growth and tooth structure. Vitamin D is necessary for transporting calcium into bone.

The sun also affects people's moods. When there is a rainy, cloudy day people stay inside and are not as easy going as they are when the sun is shinning. As soon as the sun comes out, peoples' moods start to change, and they become happy and easy going. Sunshine helps to brighten up our day. During the winter there is less sunlight, and we stay inside more, which makes us irritable and not so easy going. However, in the summer we stay outside more and people, as a whole, are friendlier. Sunlight plays an important role in this. There are many glands and organs in the body that operate directly by sunlight. The pituitary gland, which is responsible for growth and reproduction, will atrophy or decrease in size without sunlight. If you are not getting the sun's rays on your skin, start today. If you are in the sun for long periods of time, it is important that you wear protective clothing to protect the skin from sunburn. It is important to avoid the sun for long periods of time, but it is also important to expose our bodies to the sun. Even animals know not to stay in the sun for long periods of time. Cows, horses, dogs, cats, and other animals will use the sunlight in the mornings and afternoons, and during the midday, they will find shade to protect them from the heat of the sun. The sun has many great benefits to the body, and to deprive it from the sun would not make sense.

> *Ecclesiastes 11:7 Truly the light is sweet, and a pleasant thing it is for the eyes to behold the sun.*

Love

Everyone needs love. Love is a feeling of belonging to someone or something. Love is to cherish or show strong affection toward someone or something. Everyone in the world wants to be loved. When we love someone or have a feeling that we are being loved, it helps build up our immune system. It is believed that love helps build up secretory IgA levels in the body. Secretory IgA is an antibody that provides protection against bacteria, viruses, and other invading toxins in the mucus membranes. These antibodies line up along the immune system and are the first to attack invading toxins in the mucus membranes. Secretory IgA levels in the elderly population tend to be low, but when they come in contact with puppies, cats, or other playful animals, their Secretory IgA levels may increase. Pets tend to make people healthier and happier. They give us something to play with and talk to, and they don't cause much stress. Pets give much love and can help you live a healthier life. Love is the greatest force governing the world today. Without it the world will not stand. Start to show other people love and become healthy.

Laughter

Laughter is also good for the soul. It is believed that laughter helps to build up secretory IgA antibodies as well. Laughter helps to relieve stress and takes the mind and body off of problems and pain. It causes the body to relax, giving it an internal massage. Watching a comedy program on television can be a great stress releaser. Laughter helps to build up the immune system, allowing antibodies to fight off invading bacteria and viruses.[28] It is important that we keep laughter in our lives. Laughing makes us happy and plays a major role in keeping our bodies healthy. Start laughing when you hear something funny and watch your health improve. Laughter is medicine.

Proverbs 17:22 A merry heart doeth good like medicine: but a broken spirit drieth the bones.

Bowel Movements

There are many people who may call me weird for writing about this topic, but bowel movements (BMs) are very important to our health. This subject should relate to everyone who reads this book, after all, we all have them. Bowel movements should play a role in our lives everyday. Bowel movements should be relaxing and enjoyable. BMs help relax the body and relieve stress that has built up in our bodies during the day. Sometimes bowel movements are so relaxing that we play music, read books and magazines, or just take off all our clothes to enjoy them. BMs should never be a strain on the body. Some people dread having a BM because it causes them to strain, and it is painful. You should never see blood with BMs and they should never hurt. BMs play a very important role in good health because they rid the body of toxins and other wastes. We should feel happy and light after BMs.

Many people take bowel movements for granted, but there are some who don't have them as often as they should. If you eat three meals a day and don't have at least one bowel movement a day, then your GI tract is clogged. You should have bowel movements at least once a day. There are people who have BMs once a week, and they think that's normal. Some people may have BMs once a month and think that's normal. Keep in mind that these people are eating three or more meals a day. I have asked people many times if they have BMs, and they say yes, of course. I then ask how often, and many will say once a week or every other day, as if that is normal. Let's use common sense. If you put more food in your body than is coming out, then something is wrong. For example, if you have BMs everyday for a week without flushing the toilet, the toilet will begin to smell, form poisons, and the waste will decay in the toilet.

It is important to flush the toilet after each bowel movement so that we can get rid of the toxins in the toilet. I know this is a weird image, but stay with me on this. The same happens inside the body. When we don't have BMs regularly, food begins to pile up in the GI tract and release toxins and poisons in our bodies. These poisons can turn into tumors, cancers, arthritis, halitosis, and other diseases. If we were able to get rid of them through BMs, then these foods would not have time to form these diseases. Just like the toilet needs flushing every time we have a BM, our GI tract needs flushing every time we eat a heavy meal. It is very important to our health that we have bowel movements regularly. Keeping dead foods inside our bodies will only lead to sickness and disease.

How often should you have bowel movements? A person should have the same number of BMs as meals they eat each day. If you eat three full meals a day, then you should have three BMs that day. This is usually not the case with people who don't eat a majority of healthy high fiber foods that grow from the earth. People who have the same number of BMs as the meals they eat are usually people who eat only foods that grow from the earth. Since this is rare, it is important that you have, at a minimum, at least one BM a day. If you eat two or more complete meals a day with no bowel movements that day, then your system is clogged. It is important to eat foods that will clean out the GI tract and help it get rid of toxins. People who don't have BMs on a daily basis don't eat healthy, high-fiber foods in their diets. These people eat lots of meats, refined and processed foods, dairy products, and other dead foods that clog up the bowels. These foods have no fiber in them, and they just sit in the GI tract, form poisons, and cause a strain on the GI tract. The waste from these foods coming down the GI tract for elimination can cause the bowel wall to tear (fissures), form blood in the stool, and hemorrhoids in the rectum. Getting rid of foods with no fiber puts an extra load on the GI tract because the bowels do all the work. Foods that have fiber in them push their way through the bowels without the bowels doing much work. Fruits and vegetables will not cause the GI system to strain when having BMs. These foods get in and they get out.

If you are not having bowel movements at least once a day, and you are eating everyday, start to add more high fiber foods to your diet. These foods help clean out the GI tract and provide the body with lots of energy. It is normal to have BMs and to be regular, and it is very important to your health that you have them at least once a day. Foods that grow from the earth are the only foods that have live fiber in them, which assists the GI tract in eliminating waste. Reduce your stress, eat a majority of God's Original Diet, and cleanse your body. You will have regular BMs everyday and your body will get rid of toxins that could have caused diseases to form in your body.

Positive Attitude

> *Proverbs 23:7 For as a man thinketh in his heart so is he.*

A positive mental attitude is very important because if we are not positive about life, then we will certainly fail at it. Having a positive attitude means that no matter what life throws your way, you will overcome it. If a sickness or disease enters our body we have to believe that we can overcome it. If we do not believe it, then it will surely take over our body and mind. A positive mental attitude also helps us to be healthy by keeping our mind occupied with positive thinking. A positive mind is a healthy mind. If the mind is full of filth and trashy thinking, it can cause the body to become filthy and trashy. After all, the mind controls the body, which means the body is influenced by whatever the mind thinks. When your mind is occupied with positive things, you don't have time to do wrong.

The way we think can affect our health in both positive and negative ways. Our thoughts affects the body in many ways. Our body tenses up when we worry, or are fearful, depressed, angry, jealous, envious, anxious, or fill our minds with other negative thoughts. When we are tense, our muscles contract, which wastes energy and causes fatigue.

Worry, anger, depression, stress, and other toxic thinking can upset heart, kidney, liver, and other organ functions. Toxic thinking also causes headaches, fever, diarrhea, constipation, fainting, nausea, and vomiting.[29] These thoughts and feelings can also cause the GI tract to stop functioning properly. These emotional thoughts also keep you from making positive common sense decisions. They cloud the mind, often causing a person to make unhealthy and unwise decisions. This type of thinking is very destructive to the body. Positive thoughts relax the body and bring peace of mind, which allows us to make good common sense decisions. Positive thinking helps the body digest food better, helps you rest and sleep well. Thinking positively also helps you get along better with your friends and family.

Positive thinking makes the body as a whole function better. People will want to be around you and ask you for advice. If you are a negative person, start thinking positively today. Say positive things to your children, and say positive things to the people around you. Have a positive outlook on life even though everything around you may seem troublesome.

Thinking positive thoughts and saying positive words will improve your health and make your body feel great. When you start to think positive thoughts your body will become relaxed and your health will improve. When people say bad things about you, just smile at them and let it go in one ear and out the other instead of bringing anger into your body. Start today, thinking positively and saying positive things, and watch your health improve. I understand it's hard to be positive in this day and time with the world in the shape it is in. There are so many things that influence us to take a wrong path and make wrong choices in life. That is why we must keep our faith in God.

God

> *Psalms 103:3 Bless the Lord who healeth all thy diseases.*

I should have listed God as the first aspect of good health, but I saved the best for last. If we do not have faith in God, then we will fall for anything that comes along. I do not understand how some people believe that there is not a higher power looking down and controlling the world. Some people think that the world just appeared, and humans and other animals were put on this great earth. There are many man-made theories on the evolution of man, and how the world was created, but they always differ from what is found in the Bible. Man always has to think deeply to try and figure things out, when most of his problems and situations are so simple to solve.

Many people feel that if there is a God, there would not be so much violence in the world. This is far from the truth. Man controls everything that goes on in the world. Since he created the world, God has given man instructions to follow. It is up to man to follow the laws and when we do not, we must face the consequences. Our health is similar. If we do not eat a majority of foods that God told us to eat, then we may pay for it with sickness and diseases. If we pollute our planet and don't take care of our environment, then we must pay the price with global warming, drought, famine, hurricanes, tornadoes, and other forms of destruction. It is just that simple. Most things that happen on this planet happen because of man's actions, not God's.

God has given man all the instructions he needs to live a healthy and long life. It is man who causes the violence and destruction on earth, not God. So, the reason that the world is so violent is not because there is no God, it is because man has gotten away from God. Many of us suffer from problems because we do not involve God in our lives. Man brings problems upon himself; it is not God's fault.

If a father tells his son to not play with fire, and the son does so anyway and gets burned, it is not the father's responsibility that his son was burned; it was the son's fault. If the son had followed his father's instructions, he wouldn't have gotten burned. It is the same scenario with God and man.

It is up to man to follow God's rules, and if we do not, we must face the consequences of our actions. It's just that simple. Now that you know it is not God's fault that the world is in the shape it is in, we must learn to obey his rules. There is no way we can make it through life if we do not believe in a higher power that is watching over and protecting our lives. If you are in trouble, go to God and he will make a way for you. If you are sick, talk to God, and he will show you what you are doing or eating wrong. God has shown many disease sufferers the foods they should eat to fight off the disease, and they were healed. You don't need a degree or any other form of education for the Lord to teach you things. We control our own lives with the decisions that we make; it is not God's fault if we make bad decisions.

That is why it is important that we pray and ask him to lead and guide us everyday, and to help us in our decision-making. If you have not involved God in your life, start building a relationship with him today. There are many people who have problems in their lives because they are not close to God. We have started taking our problems to the psychiatrist instead of taking them to God. Man is taking the place of God. I can remember when man used to pray when he had problems, now he goes to a psychiatrist.

I am not saying that all psychiatrists are bad, because there are some good ones, but remember, they are human too. There are some problems that we go through that no man can understand, or give advice about. God is always right and will never fail. There is no cost to talk to God and you can talk to Him as long as you want; He will never look at his watch or get tired of listening. If you have gotten away from God, start going back to him today, and put your troubles in his hands. Life with him is less stressful, has fewer headaches, less worrying, and is definitely worth living.

Psalms 118:8 It is better to trust in the Lord than to put confidence in man.

VII.
FOR I AM THE LORD THAT HEALETH THEE

There are many diseases that man suffers from that can easily be avoided if only he would change his diet and lifestyle. If you look at the top 11 killers in America, most of them can be prevented, and all eleven are influenced by our diets. Our diet influences many things in our lives, including our thought process and actions. Even suicides and homicide are influenced by our diets. Many people who commit theses acts are full of drugs, alcohol, or both. The top eleven leading causes of death in American are: 1. heart disease, 2. cancer, 3. infectious diseases, 4. strokes, 5. unintentional injuries, 6. chronic obstructive lung diseases, 7. pneumonia and influenza, 8. diabetes mellitus, 9. suicide, 10. chronic liver disease and cirrhosis, and 11. homicide. Diet plays a very important role in many of these top killers. In this section I will discuss how we develop these diseases, common ways to treat them, and how we can prevent or reverse the disease process.

Obesity

Obesity is the leading contributor to many of the diseases that plague man. More than half of the population in America is obese, including our children. Obesity is not only found among humans, but it is also found in our pets today. There are several reasons why obesity occurs, and many of them have something to do with the food we eat. There are many diseases that are due to obesity such as diabetes, cancer, heart attacks, strokes, thyroid diseases, fatigue, osteoporosis, high blood pressure, tumors, high cholesterol, and many more.[1]

Obese means to be excessively fat. Being obese is like a normal weight person caring weights on his/her body. Obese people tire easily because they are carrying so much extra weight. Do you see many obese senior citizens? No. Obese people do not live as long as people who maintain a normal weight. As obese people age they are more likely to be put on some kind of medication, and their quality of life is poor.

There are many factors that play a role in obesity. Obesity can come from not eating healthy foods. When we eat excessive amounts of unhealthy food, we starve our body of nutrients. Unhealthy foods don't have any nutrients in them that the body desires, so eating these foods in excessive amounts cause the body to crave healthy foods. For example, let's say you are the typical person who eats at McDonald's,

Wendy's, Burger King, and other fast food restaurants everyday. These foods don't have any nutrients in them that your body wants, therefore after eating these foods, your body still craves nutrients.

Your stomach is full of food, but these dead foods did not meet your body's nutrient supply. As long as fast foods and other junk foods are in your diet, the body's nutrient supply will never be met. So you continue to eat, and eat, and eat, until the nutrient supply is met. At this point you are overweight, or even obese. If you continue to eat dead foods you will become obese. If you start to eat healthy foods from the earth, the body's nutrient supply will be met, and the body will feel full. You will eat less food, supply the body with proper nutrition, and at the same time, lose weight.

Another contributor to the obesity problem in America is that we put more food into our bodies than we move out of our bodies. Whenever more food enters the body than is going out the bowels expand and swell, causing obesity. When people are overweight, they eat more food than they expel through bowel movements. What causes us to eat more foods than what we expel? The major reason is that we eat unhealthy foods with no fiber in them. When you eat three or more unhealthy meals a day, you increase your chances of becoming obese.

This is why it is important to eat high fiber foods. High fiber foods go through the GI tract, cleaning up and getting rid of toxins through bowel movements. Therefore, BMs play a very important role in avoiding obesity, and eating high fiber foods are the best way to have regular BMs.

The biggest contributor to obesity is the way we prepare foods. The meats that we buy are full of hormones and antibiotics. When animals are raised for eating, their environment is so filthy that they cannot survive without being pumped full of antibiotics. Diseases are all around, such as cancer, pneumonia, heart disease, bacteria, and viruses. Hormones make these animals grow fat and fast, and are passed into our bodies when we eat them.

These hormones go to work as soon as they enter your body, causing you to become fat, very fast. They are not only found in meats that we eat, but they are also passed into cow's milk, eggs, butter, ice-creams, and other animal products we eat. The hormones from these foods, if eaten everyday in every meal, will make us fat very fast.

People who eat a majority of earth-grown foods are not obese. Eating excessive amounts of meat and animal products contribute to the obesity problem in America.

If you are obese, do you eat lots of meat and animal products? If you know someone who is obese, do they eat sweet sugary processed foods? Probably so. Do you exercise on a regular basis? Probably not.

Obesity is very simple to understand. If you want to lose weight, you have to exercise and practice the other spiritual aspects of maintaining good health. Most importantly, "eat the way God intended."

Heart and Cardiovascular Disease

Heart disease is America's number one killer and obesity plays a big role in heart disease. It takes hundreds of thousands of lives a year, both young and old. Heart disease consists of many diseases that develop in the heart. The heart is the most important muscle in the body, and most people don't take care of it.

Heart disease comes from not taking care of your heart. The two most important ways that you can take care of your heart is through diet and exercise. Of course, this is old news that we've heard before. Heart attacks, congestive heart failure, hypertension, and other heart diseases can be controlled, prevented, or resolved if we eat healthy foods and exercise the heart. The heart is a muscle that pumps blood to every organ in the body. Without the action of the heart, we die. It is important to keep your heart in good shape so that it can continue to keep you alive, because when the heart dies, you die.

Cardiovascular diseases occur in the blood vessels - the arteries and veins. Atherosclerosis, arteriosclerosis, strokes, thrombus, and embolus are the most common cardiovascular diseases. Again, diet and exercise play the most important role in preventing these illnesses. Some risk factors for heart and cardiovascular diseases are cigarette smoking, high blood cholesterol, high blood pressure, obesity, and lack of exercise. The more risk factors you have, the greater the risk for developing these diseases.

Artherosclerosis

Artherosclerosis is one of the major causes of heart and cardiovascular diseases. Artherosclerosis occurs when cholesterol, fats, and other substances build up in the walls of the arteries that supply blood to the heart and brain. This plaque clogs and narrows the arteries, slowing down and blocking the flow of blood supplying the heart and brain. One of the most important functions of blood is to carry nutrients and oxygen to the heart and brain. When oxygen and nutrients are blocked from the heart and brain due to atherosclerosis, the heart muscle is destroyed, resulting in chest pain (angina) and eventually heart attacks or death. The same happens with the brain; a buildup of atherosclerosis blocks the arteries supplying blood and oxygen to the brain and causes a transient ischemic attack and eventually a stroke.

Atherosclerosis is a slow progressive disease that usually starts early in childhood, but does not show symptoms until later in life. But how do we get atherosclerosis? Atherosclerosis is a disease that takes years to develop. Drinking cow's milk forms arteriosclerosis early in life when we start drinking cow's milk. Yes, one component of atherosclerosis is cholesterol, and when we feed our babies cow's milk, which has cholesterol in it, it can start the buildup of atherosclerosis. We then begin to eat cereals with cow's milk added. As the child grows older we begin to eat excessive amounts of meats and animal products. These foods contain cholesterol and fat, components of atherosclerosis. When we turn 40 or 50 years old, we have eaten enough animals, fats, and other dead foods to completely clog our arteries. This is when we suffer heart attacks and strokes, usually due to a buildup of atherosclerosis. If the majority of foods you eat are fats from animals, cow's milk, fried foods, processed refined foods, cigarettes, and other unhealthy foods, then atherosclerosis has probably been building up in your arteries for years. This means that the foods we feed our children will determine their health later in life.

Cigarette smoking also increases the risk of atherosclerosis.[2] Nicotine and other chemicals found in tobacco are very toxic to the blood vessel walls. So how can we reduce atherosclerosis from building up in our arteries? The answer is simple; do not eat excessive amounts of foods that make up atherosclerosis - cholesterol and saturated fat. We only get cholesterol from meats and animal products, so one way to stop atherosclerosis formation is to reduce your meat intake, or to not eat it at all.

Another way is to reduce other foods made from animal products, such as cow's milk, eggs, cheese, and other dairy products. Again, we only get saturated fat, a component of atherosclerosis, from eating meats and other animal products. Most vegetables and nuts do not contain saturated fats. The fats found in vegetables and nuts are unsaturated fats, and they do not clog up blood vessels. So, if atherosclerosis is made up of substances that come from eating animals and animal products, then it makes sense that we should reduce or eliminate those foods from our diet.

To avoid atherosclerosis exercise and engage in physical activity, start to reduce your stress level, and, most importantly, start to eat healthy foods that grow from the earth. These foods do not clog arteries and decrease blood flow. If you want to avoid atherosclerosis, which will eventually lead to heart disease and strokes, eat the way

God intended.

Heart Attacks

Heart attacks, also called myocardial infarction or MI, are the leading cause of heart disease. MI means that tissue death has occurred somewhere in the heart. When blood flow is cut off to an area of the heart, the affected area dies from lack of blood flow and oxygen. Once part of the heart dies, it will never function again. The heart is the body's hardest working organ. It continuously pumps blood through arteries to all the body's tissues. The heart also has its own supply of arteries, which supply the heart with its own supply of blood. Just like every muscle in the body, the heart needs blood to function. The arteries that supply the heart with blood are called coronary arteries.

Coronary arteries carry rich oxygenated blood to the muscular walls of the heart. If blood flow to these muscle walls are blocked a heart attack occurs. Chest pain is the most common symptom of a heart attack. Even when there is chest pain with no MI, this is a warning sign that MI is soon to come if lifestyle changes don't occur. Other common symptoms of a heart attack are sweating, and pain in the left shoulder and arm, neck or jaw. A feeling of heartburn and indigestion, nausea, and vomiting are also common symptoms. Some people describe a heart attack as a feeling as if the chest is being crushed by a heavy weight. About one and a half million Americans suffer a heart attack every year.

MI's can be fatal or they can leave the body in a chronically disabled condition, but many people have survived with only minor injuries to the heart. The prognosis for life after a heart attack depends on how severe the heart attack was. What causes a heart attack? There are many reasons people have heart attacks, such as fear, stress, and a decreased oxygen supply to the heart, but the most common reason is our diet. In most cases of myocardial infarctions, the restriction of blood flow to the heart results from atherosclerosis. Atherosclerosis is made up of cholesterol, fats, and other particles, which the body stores in the walls of arteries when they are in large supply. This cholesterol plaque slowly thickens over time, narrowing the arteries.

As the arteries begin to narrow, less blood flows to the heart, until the artery is completely blocked - and you suffer a heart attack. When we eat a lot of cholesterol and fatty foods, our body has to store fatty plaque somewhere until it has time to get rid of it. For some odd reason the body stores it in the major arteries which supply the heart and brain. The body will get rid of cholesterol and fats, if given the opportunity.

However, most people eat meat and animal products everyday, three times a day, therefore, the body does not have time to get rid of cholesterol and fat because it is constantly digesting new food coming into the body. Cholesterol is not found in fruits, vegetables, nuts, seeds, or grains, therefore they cannot cause a high cholesterol level in the blood. The fats found in these foods are essential for the body. The answer is very simple; people who have heart attacks eat fast foods, lots of heavy meats, dairy products, and other unhealthy foods. If you have suffered a heart attack and don't wish to suffer another, you have to change your eating habits. The reason so many people have a second and third heart attacks is because they didn't change their lifestyles between attacks. Most doctors tell their patients to go on a high fiber, low-cholesterol diet after suffering heart attacks, but never tell them what foods contain fiber and cholesterol. Sometimes it is not enough to give up red meats; sometimes you need to give up all meats, no matter what color. It is also wise to give up coffee, tea, soda, and cigarettes.

Start to eat a majority of foods that grow from the earth. Start to reduce meats and animal products from your diet. Exercise on a regular basis and reduce your stress levels. If you practice these simple rules you will start strengthening your heart and prevent cholesterol and fatty clots from forming inside your arteries, thus preventing a heart attack.

High Blood Pressure

High blood pressure, also called hypertension, is a risk factor for many heart and cardiovascular diseases and is very common in America. It is estimated that about one out of every four Americans has high blood pressure. Obesity plays a major role in high blood pressure. Hypertension contributes to hundreds of thousands of deaths a year. When the heart beats, it pumps blood through the entire body. The blood delivers nutrients such as vitamins and minerals to different muscles, glands, bones, and other structures of the body. When high blood pressure occurs, the small blood vessels called arterioles constricts, or narrow, which causes the blood to exert excessive pressure against the blood vessel walls. When blood vessels narrow, the heart pumps harder than normal to maintain an adequate blood supply throughout the body, thus causing high blood pressure.

This excessive pressure can eventually cause the heart to enlarge and damage muscle tissues, which causes the heart to fail (congestive heart failure). It can damage the blood vessel walls, leading to heart attacks and strokes, and put excessive work on the kidneys, leading to kidney disease.³ In fact, high blood pressure contributes to about 75% of all strokes and heart disease.⁴ Chronic hypertension is associated with memory deterioration in older people, such as reduced memory and attention span, Alzheimer's disease, and dementia.⁵ It can also lead to arteriosclerosis and kidney damage.

Blood pressure is the force of the blood pushing against the walls of the arteries and is measured in millimeters of mercury in two numbers. The first pressure measurement, or the top number, is taken when the heart contracts which is called systolic pressure - this is when the heart is pumping. The second pressure measurement, or the bottom number, is taken between contractions of the heart, which is called diastolic - this is when the heart relaxes. Although the ideal blood pressure is 120/80, every individual's normal blood pressure is different, meaning that just because one person's blood pressure is normal at 120/80 does not mean that the next person should be the same. People are not considered to have high BP until it reads 140/90 and above. If your blood pressure is between 120/80 and 139/89, you are considered normal to high normal. Your blood pressure does not have to be between these two measurements to be normal. It is possible to have a normal blood pressure lower than 120/80.

In fact, most endurance or long distance runners have a blood pressure lower than 120/80, because their hearts have adjusted to their lifestyle of running. We should try, however, to keep our blood pressure around the average normal of 120/80 or lower.

What causes high blood pressure? There are two types of hypertension - essential hypertension that doctors are unable to identify a cause for, and secondary hypertension that is caused by other factors. There are many things that can cause secondary hypertension. The first major cause is atherosclerosis.

Atherosclerosis clogs up arteries and causes the heart to pump blood throughout the body harder than normal. As atherosclerosis begins to form in the arteries, it blocks blood flow to major organs of the body. As these arteries become blocked, the heart works harder than normal just to supply an adequate amount of blood to the rest of the body. As this process continues, it leads to high blood pressure.

Another major cause of hypertension is obesity. Obesity plays a major role in the pumping action of the heart. As your body weight increases, your blood pressure rises. The more weight a person carries, the harder the heart has to work. So the majority of people with high blood pressure are usually overweight. There are legal drugs that also cause hypertension, such as aspirin and Ibuprofen, if used in excessive amounts. Hypertension is seen in people who consume at least three or more alcoholic drinks a day, caffeine drinkers, and smokers.

Stress plays a major role in hypertension as well. Stress causes muscles to tense and contract, causing the blood pressure to rise. Excessive blood pressure in the brain can lead to headaches, nausea, drowsiness, confusion, and loss of vision. Eating lots of heavy meats raises the blood pressure. The heart has to send extra blood to the GI tract so that it can digest these foods putting extra work load on the heart.

How can we prevent high blood pressure? There are many things that can be done to prevent high blood pressure. The best way to prevent or decrease hypertension is to maintain a healthy weight, by eating healthy foods. Eating food that grows from the earth keeps the GI tract clean and takes waste out of the body. They are easy to digest and provide lots of energy, which means less work for the heart, less pressure in the blood vessel walls, and normal blood pressure. Another way to lower blood pressure is to become active. Most people with hypertension are not active. It is important to exercise the body to strengthen it. Being physically active can reduce your risk for heart disease, help lower cholesterol and high blood pressure. Walking and running are great ways to reduce or prevent high blood pressure because when you sweat, you get rid of toxins through the pores of your skin. Walking and running help strengthen the heart, which protects from heart disease. Other physical activities such as jumping rope and swimming strengthen the heart as well.

Sunlight has been shown to reduce blood pressure. Studies have proven that exposing the body to the sun helps lower blood pressure.[6] Sun rays help relax the heart, so try to get five to ten minutes of sunlight a day, preferably in the early morning or late afternoon when the rays of the sun are more comfortable.

Another way to prevent or control high blood pressure is to reduce or eliminate the use of salt. Table salt is terrible on the heart and kidneys, and many people with hypertension, can lower their blood pressure when they stop using it. Reduce your meat intake. Meat causes the heart to work extra hard and is terrible on the kidneys as well. Stop drinking caffeine, alcohol, and smoking cigarettes. Reduce your stress levels, by meditating and relaxing. Start to add more fruits, vegetables, whole grains, and raw nuts and seeds to your diet. These foods are high in fiber and give the body plenty of energy. Eating earth grown foods is less stressful on the heart, which decreases blood pressure.

Strokes

Strokes are the same as heart attacks; the only difference is that strokes occur in the brain. People at risk for strokes are usually older adults who eat an unhealthy diet, don't exercise, and whose lives are full of added stress. People with high blood pressure, obese people, smokers, and diabetics are also at risk. People in the southeastern states have the highest risk for stroke than any other area in the country. Southeastern states also have the highest death rate from strokes than any other area of the country. In fact, southeastern states have such high rates of stroke, among people of all races and both sexes, that they are called the "Stroke Belt States" - Alabama, Georgia, Arkansas, Tennessee, North and South Carolina, Indiana, Kentucky, Louisiana, Virginia, and of course, my home state, Mississippi.

In the southeast we eat everything on the hog, from the brain to the tail. Nothing goes to waste. When a person suffers a stroke, brain tissue is damaged due to a lack of blood flow to a particular part of the brain. Strokes are often caused by a blood clot in an artery narrowed by atherosclerosis, but can be caused by a tear in the artery as well. The amount of time it takes to recover from a stroke depends on the damage done during a stroke, and where in the brain the stroke occurred. Blood is supplied to the brain through two main arteries - the vertebral and carotid arteries.

The carotid arteries supply the brain with blood through the front of the neck and the vertebral arteries connect to form the basilar artery and supply the brain with blood through the rear of the neck. The brain needs a constant supply of oxygen to function and control the body. The brain uses about 25% of the body's oxygen supply but cannot store it, so the body has to keep the brain supplied with it at all times. A reduction of oxygen to the brain for a very short period of time can be deadly, leading to strokes. A stroke should always be taken seriously, whether it is light or major. Light strokes, also called transient ischemic attacks (TIA's), are usually a warning sign that a major stroke is on the way if the person does not change his or her lifestyle. Unlike other cells in the body, cells in the brain do not repair or regenerate themselves, meaning that when the cells in the brain die, that part of the brain is dead forever.

The results of strokes can be detrimental. Many stroke survivors have to retrain themselves to walk, talk, write, and do other simple tasks that most people take for granted. If blood is blocked from supplying the area of the brain that controls walking and balance, then after a stroke, that person will not be able to walk. If blood is blocked from supplying the area of the brain that controls speech, then after a stroke, that person will not be able to talk. Strokes affect the brain, which affects the nerves of the body. When the nerves in a certain area of the body are affected by a stroke, that part of the body no longer functions. There are two types of strokes and they are named based on how the stroke occurs. If a stroke occurs due to atherosclerosis, it is called an ischemic stroke, due to a lack of oxygen and blood flow to the brain. If the stroke occurred due to a tear in the artery, it is called a hemorrhagic stroke, due to bleeding.

Eighty percent of all strokes are ischemic strokes. These strokes are usually caused by a thrombus or an embolus in the brain. A thrombus is a blood clot that forms within one of the brain's arteries. A thrombotic stroke usually occurs when an artery that supplies the brain with blood is blocked by a clot that forms as a result of atherosclerosis, also called hardening of the arteries. An embolus is a blood clot formed elsewhere in the body that travels through the bloodstream and eventually lodges in an artery in the brain, blocking oxygen and blood flow to that part of the brain.

Most hemorrhagic strokes occur due to high blood pressure and atherosclerosis. The heart has to pump blood harder than normal just to supply the body with a sufficient amount of blood and oxygen when the arteries are blocked by fat. These excessively hard pumps by the heart cause extra pressure to build up in the arteries of the brain. The heart pumps the blood so hard through the blood vessels that it causes the blood vessel walls to tear, resulting in a stroke. High blood pressure contributes to about 70% of all strokes.

Heavy alcohol use and drinking coffee, tea, and other caffeine drinks also increase the risk for a stroke. These drugs raise the blood pressure and, if atherosclerosis is present, can cause a stroke.

The majority of strokes are usually caused by atherosclerosis and this fatty artery plugger only comes from eating unhealthy dead fatty foods. If you know someone who has had a stroke, do they eat dead fatty foods such as excessive amounts of meats, dairy products, French fries, potato chips, and fried foods? Do they love to drink coffee, tea, sodas, and smoke cigarettes? Do they have lots of stress in their life? Probably so. If you know someone who has suffered from a stroke, do they eat a majority of the foods that grow from the earth? Do they exercise regularly by walking or running? Do they cope with stressful situations well? Probably not. Start to include healthy foods in your diet. Eat high fiber foods that grow from the earth. These foods fight against strokes, they don't cause them.

High Blood Cholesterol

High blood cholesterol has been confusing many people for years. Every year we hear that some foods are good to eat, and the next year they are bad. Cholesterol plays a major role in our health. It is a normal substance found in the muscles and other tissues of the body. Cholesterol is a lipid, or fat-like substance that is critical to good health. Cholesterol is used throughout the body and is converted into various hormones, such as bile and vitamin D. There are two sources of cholesterol - cholesterol formed naturally in the liver and cholesterol found in our diet. Cholesterol is found only in animals, meaning that we can only get cholesterol through our diet from eating meats, and other animal products, such as dairy products, and eggs. All animals produce cholesterol in their bodies naturally just as humans do.

Cholesterol is measured by the amount of lipids or fat found in the blood. A cholesterol level above 200 is considered high. If your blood cholesterol level is high, you are at great risk of suffering a heart attack or stroke. Cholesterol is not found in foods that grow from the earth. If we eat a majority of healthy foods that grow from the earth, chances are, your blood cholesterol level is normal. As long as the liver produces cholesterol without high levels coming into the body from our diets then our cholesterol levels will remain normal.

Cholesterol becomes a problem to our health when we put excessive amounts of it into the body through our diet. When we eat lots of meats and other animal products, cholesterol is constantly coming into the body. High blood cholesterol is a major contributor to heart disease and stroke. Cholesterol is transported to muscles and other tissues of the body by the blood, but unlike most nutrients, cholesterol needs special carriers, and these carriers are called lipoproteins. Two lipoproteins make the news when it comes to high blood cholesterol - the bad cholesterol carrier, low-density lipoprotein (LDL) and high-density lipoprotein (HDL), the good cholesterol carrier.

LDL is the major cholesterol carrier in the blood. Excessive amounts build up in the blood vessel walls with other substances and form atherosclerosis, which restricts the flow of blood to the heart and brain, resulting in a heart attack or a stroke. HDL carries about 25% of the cholesterol from the muscles back to the liver. It also cleans the cholesterol that the LDL may leave behind in the arteries. It is important that we have high amounts of HDL in our bloodstream to help keep our blood cholesterol levels normal. Fats also play a major role in our cholesterol levels and the three major fats that affect cholesterol levels are saturated, unsaturated, and trans fats.

Most saturated fats come from animals and animal products. Meats, eggs, cheeses, ice cream, butter, and other animal products contain high amounts of saturated fats. Studies show that saturated fats raise our blood cholesterol level more than any other foods we eat. Trans fats come from liquid vegetable oils that are processed and used as cooking fats. Vegetable oils are made under a process called hydrogenation which heats and processes the oil. Hydrogenation changes the structure of unsaturated fat to saturated fat - the same fat found in meats.

Trans fat increases the risk of a heart attack by raising blood levels of LDL, and lowering HDL, which clogs the arteries. In fact, studies are showing that trans fats may be even worse for your heart than saturated fats found in animals. Trans fats are found in margarine, hydrogenated vegetable shortening, processed peanut butter, many fried foods, cookies, cakes, pies, crackers, potato chips, and other common processed foods.

Unsaturated fats can help lower cholesterol levels. These fats are found in foods that grow from the earth. Of course, they will lower cholesterol levels in the blood because they have no cholesterol in them. There are two types of unsaturated fats - monounsaturated and polyunsaturated. Monounsaturated fats are found in foods from plants, including olive, peanut and canola oil. They help lower bad cholesterol levels (LDL) in the blood. Polyunsaturated fats are found in foods from plants, including safflower, sunflower, soybean, and corn oil. These fats help lower LDL in the blood.

So how do we lower our cholesterol levels? It is very simple. Start to include more fruits and vegetables in your diet. Vegetables and fruit help clean unwanted fats, clots, and other harmful substances out of the arteries. Reduce your intake of animal and dairy products. This is the only way we get excess cholesterol in the body, so it makes sense that this is how our blood cholesterol levels are elevated. Start to exercise; do brisk walking, swimming or cycling. Sunlight also helps lower cholesterol levels in the blood.[7] When the sun's rays stimulate the skin, the cholesterol found under the skin is converted into vitamin D, which helps lower cholesterol. So try to get five to ten minutes of sunlight a day, preferably in the early morning or late evening when the rays of the sun are more comfortable.

Reduce your meat and dairy intake, and if possible, eliminate it. Reduce the amount of fatty foods you eat such as margarine, potato chips, cookies, cakes, pies, and other processed foods. If you smoke, make up your mind to stop. Cigarette smoking increases the bad cholesterol, LDL, and decreases the good cholesterol, HDL, levels in the blood, and also constricts the arteries. If you have high blood cholesterol, do you eat excessive amounts of meat everyday? If you know someone with high blood cholesterol, do they eat butter, margarine, eggs, dairy products and other animal food products? Do they eat potato chips, cookies, cakes, pies, and other fatty foods? Do they smoke tobacco? Are they overweight? Probably so. Do they eat a majority of foods that come from the earth, especially fruits and vegetables? Do they exercise on a regular basis, especially walking and running? Do they keep a low level of stress in their lives? Probably not. If you want to lower your cholesterol, start to eat healthy foods. Foods from the earth will slow fatty buildup in the walls of the arteries and reduce your blood cholesterol levels.

Heartburn

Heartburn is not associated with the heart at all, because it only involves the stomach and the lower portion of the esophagus. Heartburn is a pain felt in the stomach due to the build up of stomach acid. This acid backs up into the esophagus, a tube of muscle that connects the throat to the stomach, and causes a burning feeling in the esophagus. The esophagus is alongside the heart, which is why the burning feeling feels as if it is in the heart. Thus, we get the term heartburn. Other terms for heartburn are gastroesophagel reflux disease and acid indigestion. Antacids are commonly used to relieve heartburn. It is estimated that more than 60 million American adults experience heartburn at least once a month, and about 25 million adults suffer from heartburn on a daily basis. About 25% of pregnant women experience daily heartburn, and about 50% of pregnant women experience heartburn when under stress.

Heartburn is described as feeling as if food is coming back up into the mouth, leaving an acid and bitter taste. Heartburn can last for hours at a time and is often worse after eating. There are a few long-term complications of heartburn, such as esophagitis, which occurs due to excess stomach acid in the esophagus. If acid stays in the esophagus for long periods of time it can burn through the esophagus and cause esophageal bleeding or ulcers.

Narrowing of the esophagus may occur from heartburn as well. Heartburn can also destroy the lining of the esophagus, which may eventually lead to cancer. Some people may have surgery for heartburn. These surgeries usually increase the pressure in the lower esophagus to stop the backflow of acid into the esophagus.

Where does heartburn come from, and how can we prevent it? The answer is very simple. Eating heavy meals will cause heartburn. The stomach becomes full and acid buildup begins to flow back into the esophagus. Lying down immediately after a meal will cause heartburn. This is why it is important to eat two to three hours before resting.

Being overweight will increase heartburn, but the majority of heartburn comes from the foods that we eat. It is common for us to eat acid-forming foods which cause heartburn. When we eat excessive amounts of foods that have to be broken down by acid, we usually suffer from heartburn. Foods that are acid-forming are meats, dairy products, fried foods, alcohol, coffee, sodas, cigarettes, and other man-made foods.

Humans are alkaline species, meaning that the foods we eat should be digested by alkaline juices in the stomach and not acid. Humans have very little acid in the stomach because we only need enough to breakdown nuts, seeds, and some vegetables, not pigs, cows, and other heavy meats. When we eat excessive amounts of meats, dairy products, fried foods, alcohol and caffeine drinks, and smoke cigarettes, the stomach secretes more acid than it should normally produce. Over a long period of time, this acid can build up in the stomach and cause a backflow into the esophagus, causing heartburn.

If you suffer from heartburn, do you eat excessive amounts of meats, dairy products, fried, and fatty foods? The answer is probably yes. If you know someone who suffers from heartburn, do they smoke cigarettes and drink coffee, sodas, Kool-aid, and alcoholic beverages? Probably so. Do they eat plenty of fruits and vegetables? Probably not. Do they drink plenty of water and exercise regularly? Probably not. Changing your diet is usually enough to stop heartburn. If it sounds too good to be true, try it for a day. Eat fruits and vegetables for a day, and your heartburn will improve.

Lung Cancer

More people die from lung cancer than any other cancer. Annually there are approximately 172,000 cases of lung cancer diagnosed with about 160,000 of those cases ending in death. There are two types of cancer that occur in the lung - large or small cell lung cancer. Large cell lung cancer, also called squamous cell carcinoma or adenocarcinoma, tend to occur in the bronchi of the lungs and people who have this type of cancer have a better survival rate than people with small cell lung cancer. Large cell lung cancer is more common than small cell lung cancer and it also grows and spreads more slowly. Small cell lung cancer is less common, but grows and spreads to other organs in the body more quickly than large cell lung cancer. Symptoms of lung cancer are a cough that does not go away and gets worse over time, constant chest pain, coughing up blood, shortness of breath, fatigue, weight loss, loss of appetite, wheezing, or hoarseness. Lung cancer spreads to the bone and brain in its final stages. Lung cancer is diagnosed through a biopsy, the examination of a sample of lung tissue under a microscope. But how can you prevent lung cancer? Lung cancer can be prevented most of the time, because most lung cancer comes from tobacco smoking.

Tobacco exposure is the most dominant risk factor for lung cancer. Tobacco smoking causes 90% of the lung cancer in males and 80% in females.[8] The most effective way to avoid lung cancer is to not use tobacco. Cigarettes contain over 3000 different harmful chemicals that damage the cells of the lungs.[9] These chemicals include carbon monoxide, ammonia, methanol, formaldehyde, and nicotine, making tobacco arguably the most addictive drug that exists - legal or illegal. What determines if a smoker has a chance of developing lung cancer depends on the age the person started smoking, how long the person has smoked, how deeply the person inhales the smoke into his/her lungs, and how many cigarettes they smoke a day. When a person stops smoking, they greatly reduce their risk for developing lung cancer. Cigar and pipe smokers also have a higher risk for developing lung cancer. People who smoke cigars, pipes, and cigarettes have a higher risk for developing mouth, larynx, throat, and other types of cancer as well.

People who breathe in second-hand smoke have a higher chance of developing lung cancer.[10] Exposure to radon gas and asbestos also causes lung cancer. Radon is an invisible, odorless, tasteless, radioactive gas that is naturally found in soil and rocks. People who work in mines may be exposed to it, and in some parts of the country, radon is found in homes. If you smoke tobacco and work around radon, your chance of developing lung cancer increases. Asbestos is a group of minerals that occur naturally as fibers and are used in industries, such as shipbuilding, mining, insulation materials, and brake repair. When asbestos is inhaled, its particles can get trapped in the lungs, damaging cells and increasing the risk for lung cancer. If you smoke and work in an environment around asbestos, your chance for developing lung cancer increases. If people would take charge of their health, lung cancer could be prevented.

Many of our teenagers are pressured into smoking cigarettes and other drugs by their peers. Cigarette companies target children, trying to get them hooked on their drug as early in life as possible. The sooner they are hooked, the more money the cigarette companies will make from your kids. They tell children that smoking is cool, and it is a way to have a good time. It keeps the weight off and keeps the body slim and trim. They paint a really pretty picture so that you will give in, and try it. That pretty picture does not show the end of your life. They do not show the gasping for air and oxygen, because cancer has eaten up your lungs, making it difficult to breath. They do not show the coughing up of blood, because cancer has destroyed your lungs. They do not show the lack of energy, because cigarettes deplete the body's energy supply. The best way to prevent lung cancer is to quit, or never start smoking. The sooner a person quits, the better chance he/she has of avoiding lung cancer. Although diet is rarely linked to lung cancer, it is important to eat live foods that grow from the earth, exercise regularly, and keep stress to a minimum. If you have or know someone with lung cancer do they smoke or are they around tobacco smoke? Probably so. A person rarely develops lung cancer without some history of tobacco smoking.

Breast Cancer

Breast cancer is probably the most feared disease among women. When most women are diagnosed with breast cancer they assume their life is over. Few manage to strike up enough willpower to fight it. Breast cancer is the second most common form of cancer among women in the U.S., and the second leading cause of cancer deaths among women. It is the leading cause of death for women between the ages of 40 and 55. It is estimated that one in nine American women will be diagnosed with breast cancer during their lifetime and about 40,000 women in the U.S. will die annually from it. Breast cancer is not just found in women. It is found in men also. About 1300 cases of breast cancer in men are reported every year.

About 400 men in the U.S. die each year from breast cancer.[11] Breast cancer is a malignant or life-threatening tumor that can develop in one or both breast. These cancers can eventually spread through the blood to other organs of the body such as the brain, bones, and heart, which can be fatal. The breast is made of fatty and fibrous connective tissue. Cancerous tumors form on these fatty tissues and begin to grow in excessive amounts, leading to lumps and bumps in the tissues of the breast. Most doctors feel that early detection of breast cancer is the best way to fight against it. The best line of defense that doctors have against this is the mammogram.

Mammograms are used to detect tumor growth in the breast tissue, but when doctors find tumors growing on the breast, then what? In most cases doctors recommend that the tumor be removed or the breast be removed. They call this preventing breast cancer. Prevention is teaching the patient how to change her lifestyle to keep cancer from growing in her body in the first place. If a mammogram detects cancer in the breast, then it was not prevented. If lifestyle changes are not made, then the cancer will just spread to another organ. How often does a person have cancer in one organ, have the organ removed, and been told they were cancer free, only to learn later the cancer spread to another organ? Many times. That means the cancer was not cured or prevented.

Women, you don't just happen to get breast cancer; there is something that you do to develop cancer inside the breast. Breast cancer is found in a majority of women who don't exercise. A number of studies show that regular exercise may lower a woman's risk for breast cancer.[12] Heavy alcohol consumption, over three drinks a week, increases the risk for cancer.[13]

Weight plays a role in breast cancer.[14] Many women who have breast cancer are overweight. The most important factor contributing to breast cancer is diet. Fats and meat play a major role in developing breast cancer, or any other kind of cancer.[15] Remember, the breast is made up of fatty tissue, and what better place for the body to deposit excessive fat, from foods we consume, than in fatty tissue. As the body deposits excess fat from the diet in breast tissue, it grows until it becomes a tumor, eventually leading to cancer. We all know that fruits and vegetables contain nutrients - phytochemicals, vitamins, and antioxidants - that help fight against cancer. What cancer-fighting nutrients do meat, alcohol, and fried fatty foods contain? None. In fact, they help contribute to the formation of cancer.

Tumors don't just happen to appear in the breast, something has to allow them to grow there over time. If you think that eating foods that are cooked over smoke, or barbecued, and fried in grease won't give you cancer and fatty tumors, think again. We already know that smoking causes cancer, so what is the difference between smoking cigarettes and eating foods with smoke inside them? Not much. Studies show that charcoal browned, fried, smoked and barbecued meats gives off a chemical called heterocyclic amines, which is known to be a cancer- causing agent.

Nitrates, another cancer-forming chemical, are found in smoked, salted, and pickled foods. Therefore, the more of these foods you eat the greater your chances are for developing breast and other cancers.[16] If you want to prevent breast cancer, start to eat more life-giving foods that grow from the earth. God has given these foods nutrients that fight against cancers, not promote them. Fats found in olive, peanut, and canola oils have been found to be protective against breast cancer. Soybeans help protect against excessive breast cell growth.[17] Tomatoes contains more phytochemicals than any other food and help fight against cancer every time you eat them. Tomatoes also contain lycopene, a nutrient that has been found to shrink breast tumors.[18] All fruits, vegetables, nuts, and seeds help fight off cancers and promote a better quality of life.

Women who breast-feed have a lower rate of developing breast cancer than women who don't.[19] So, if you want to prevent breast cancer, start to exercise more, by walking or running at least 2 to 3 times a week. If you smoke, stop. Reduce your fried, barbecued, and fatty meat intake. Reduce your intake of dairy products. If you can, stop eating them altogether. Start eating live foods from the earth. All fruits, all vegetables, all raw seeds and nuts help fight against breast cancer?

Prostate Cancer

Prostate cancer is probably the most feared cancer among men. We are taught to get our prostate checked when we turn 40 years of age. Prostate cancer is the leading cancer among men, with lung cancer being second. Prostate cancer strikes all races, young and old, but is more prevalent in the African American community. It is estimated that about 185,000 American men are diagnosed with prostrate cancer each year, and about 39,000 die from it. The prostate is a male sex gland, made of fatty tissue, which is about the size of a walnut. It is located between the bladder and the rectum and wraps around the urethra, the tube that carries urine from the bladder out through the penis. The prostate produces semen, a thick fluid that helps move sperm through the urethra and out the penis during the ejaculation stage of sex. This thick fluid covers and protects the sperm in the vagina of the female and helps it penetrate the female egg. Since the prostrate is located in front of the rectum, a doctor can check the size of the prostate by inserting a rubber-gloved finger into the rectum.

Another more preferable test is done by monitoring the blood levels of a substance called prostate specific antigen, or PSA, which, when elevated, may indicate the presence of prostate cancer. What is prostate cancer? Prostate cancer is a malignant tumor that arises in the prostate gland and can eventually spread through the blood and lymph fluid to other organs, bones, and tissues. Prostate cancer is slow growing and usually does not spread. In fact, more men die with prostate cancer than from it. Prostate cancer occurs mostly in men over the age of 40. Common signs and symptoms of prostate tumors are frequent urination, especially late at night, difficulty urinating, pain or burning during urination, inability to urinate, interrupted urination, blood in the urine, and painful sex.

Prostate cancer can be treated by surgery, which involves removal of the tumor by radiation treatment, or radical prostatectomy, removal of the prostate. These treatments have many side effects, including impotence, incontinence, and lack of pleasurable sexual activity. Some men also have their testicles removed during prostate surgery, because the testicles have been shown to produce male hormones, which may fuel prostate cancer. All these treatments can be avoided if men would change their eating habits.

Diet plays the most important role in developing prostate cancer. For example, Asian men outside the U.S. have a lower incidence of prostate cancer than Asian men who live in America. African Americans have a high incidence of prostate cancer in America, but in Africa, where they eat a majority of food that grows from the earth, prostate cancer is almost unheard of.[20] This proves that the western American Diet is the root of many of the diseases that we face. Animal fats and fried fatty foods increase the risk of developing prostate cancer. Men who eat high fatty diets - meats, fried foods, margarines, dairy products, etc. - have a higher rate of prostate cancer than those who eat foods low in fat and rich in foods that grow from the earth.[21] Again, fruits, vegetables, raw nuts, seeds, and grains help fight against all cancers, including prostate cancer. Tomatoes, and other fresh fruits, onions, garlic, broccoli, cauliflower, carrots, soybeans, and dark vegetables are great cancer fighters. It is also believed that vitamins A, D, C and E protect against prostate cancer. Fruits and vegetables are the best sources of these vitamins, and the sun provides the best source of vitamin D. In fact, states in the southern half of the U.S., where the sun shines brighter and longer, have lower prostate cancer rates than any other parts of the country.[22] Exercise also plays a major role in preventing prostate cancer.

Many men with prostate cancer eat unhealthy foods and don't exercise. If you have prostate cancer, do you eat lots of meat, dairy products, fried, and fatty foods? Probably so. If you know someone with prostate cancer, are they obese? Probably so. Do the majority of their diets include fruits and vegetables? Do they exercise on a regular basis? Probably not. If you want to prevent your chances of prostate cancer, start to eat the way God intended.

Colorectal Cancer

Colorectal cancer is among the most common cancer in the U.S. It occurs in both men and women and is usually found in people who are over the age of 50 but can occur at much younger ages. Annually approximately 130,000 men and women are diagnosed with colorectal cancer and approximately 56,000 die from this disease.

The colon and rectum are parts of the digestive system and make up the majority of the large intestine. Their function is to remove water and other nutrients from food, and to store waste from digested foods until it is ready to be passed out of the body.

The colon makes up about the first 6 feet of large intestine, and the rectum, which is the last part of the colon, measures about 8 to 10 inches. In fact, the digestive tract as a whole, from the tongue to the anus, measures the same length of a tennis court. This allows food to stay in our GI tract for long periods of time, and in many cases, what we put in our GI tract will determine how healthy it will be. A change in bowel habits such as diarrhea, constipation, or feeling that the bowel is not completely empty after a bowel movement are common symptoms of colorectal cancer. Blood in the stool, stools that are narrower than the normal, bloating, cramping, gas pains, vomiting, lower abdominal discomfort, and weight loss for no known reason are all common signs of colorectal cancer.[23] People who already have another form of cancer - women who have a history of ovarian, uterine, or breast cancer, and men who have prostate cancer - have an increased chance of developing colorectal cancer.

The major risk factor for developing colorectal cancer is a person's diet. Colorectal cancer, like most cancers, seems to be associated with diets that are high in fat and calories and low in fiber.[24] Colorectal cancer, like most cancers, seems to be diagnosed in people who don't exercise. There are many treatments for colorectal cancer but none help prevent cancer. Surgery is a common method of choice for many patients. In surgery the tumor is removed along with a healthy piece of colon or rectum. In most cases the doctor can reconnect the healthy portions of the colon and rectum, but when the healthy portions cannot be reconnected, a colostomy is done.

A colostomy is a surgical opening, also called a stoma, through the wall of the abdomen into the colon. The colon is placed outside the abdominal wall so that waste does not collect inside the body. After a patient has a colostomy, they have to wear a special bag to collect body waste, and they no longer have normal bowel movements. Chemo and radiation therapy are used to treat colorectal cancer. Even after going through all these treatments, it is possible for cancer to reappear, if the patient does not change their lifestyle.

The main cause for colorectal cancer is diet. If you eat excessive amounts of dead diseased foods, you become diseased. Doctors have already told us that colorectal cancer comes from eating high fat, low fiber foods. The foods that God intended for us to eat are high in fiber and low in fat. Fruits, vegetables, raw nuts, seeds, and whole grains all contain fiber and are low in fat, and the fats that they do provide, are needed by the body. The fiber from these foods goes throughout our GI tract and cleans out waste and other unwanted products. These foods fight against colorectal cancer, not cause it. These foods give our body energy, not take energy out of the body. If you want to prevent colorectal cancer, start to eat the way God intended. Reduce your meat and fatty food intake, and, if possible, stop eating them altogether. Start eating live foods that grow from the earth, start to drink plenty of water, start to exercise on a regular basis, and watch your chance of developing colorectal cancer decrease.

Other Cancers

There are plenty of cancers that could be prevented if only we would change our diet, by eating the way God intended. Other common cancers that could be prevented by improving our diet are urinary bladder, kidney, ovarian, testicular, throat, uterine, and endometrial cancers. Cancer can form in every organ of the body, and it is up to us to give our organs the best fuel, or proper foods, to fight against cancer. If you do not give the body the best fuel to perform its daily activities, in the end, you may develop diseases like cancer. Cancer of the bladder, throat, larynx, cervix, testicles, and even leukemia can usually be linked to smoking, diet, and lack of exercise.[25] We are eating too much meat, fried foods, dairy products, and fatty foods. We are drinking too many alcoholic beverages and caffeine drinks. We are smoking too many cigarettes, cigars, pipes, and other drugs. We are eating too much salt, sugar, artificial sweeteners, and other stimulating drugs. And when the doctor diagnose cancer, we wonder how we got it. You cannot expect a healthy body if the majority of your diet consist of unhealthy foods. You should not expect to have a healthy body if you smoke cigarettes and drink alcohol. The only way you can have a healthy body is to eat healthy life-giving foods, and live a healthy lifestyle.

Arthritis

Arthritis is the leading cause of disability in the U.S. and limits the activity of more than 7 million Americans. Millions of dollars are spent on treating and managing arthritis every year. More than 40 million Americans suffer from some form of arthritis, and it is estimated that by the year 2020, about 60 million Americans will have arthritis, and 11 million will be disabled from it. One out of every seven Americans suffers from arthritis, so chances are you have, or know someone who has, arthritis. Arthritis can occur at any age, but it is more prevalent in people over the ages of 45 to 50. Arthritis is a disease that is considered a normal part of aging. Often doctors tell us that arthritis is a disease that we have to learn to live with, that we just have to learn to put up with the pain.

Arthritis is not a disease that you have to live with, and there are ways of preventing it. Arthritis is inflammation of a joint that causes pain and loss of movement in the joint. Arthritis can become so severe that common everyday activities become difficult, such as dressing, getting in and out of bed, walking, and climbing stairs. Any joint of the body can be affected by arthritis.

Inflammation is the body's protective response to an injury or infection. During an inflammatory phase, the body produce redness, heat, pain, and swelling in an attempt to fight off and kill viruses, bacteria, and other micro-organisms that shouldn't be in the body. This is the body's natural response. But with arthritis, instead of fighting off invading organisms, the body begins to destroy itself, for reasons that many don't yet understand. What is known is that arthritis is seen in mostly people who are obese and don't exercise.

Another common substance of arthritis is uric acid, which we get from excessive amounts of meat, fried foods, and processed, refined foods.[26] Arthritis usually begins with slight morning stiffness in a particular joint, and over time, can become worse, to the point of causing its victim to become crippled or disabled. Crippled and disabled people use canes, walkers, and have hip joint replacements to allow some movement of the body. There are many kinds of arthritis that affect connective tissue, tendons, ligaments, skin, heart, lungs, eyes, and internal organs in the GI tract. There are three major forms of arthritis that many suffer from - osteoarthritis, rheumatoid arthritis, and gout.

Osteoarthritis, also known as the "wear and tear" arthritis and degenerative joint disease (DJD), results from the destruction of cartilage and other tissues in a joint. DJD is the most common type of arthritis, affecting more than 16 millions Americans. It is very common in people over the age of 65, but can affect people at a much younger age. It is also the most common form of arthritis found among athletes. DJD is caused by the breakdown or wearing away of cartilage, which is the cushion that covers the ends of bones that form joints.

DJD begins when cartilage breaks down in a joint leaving the two opposing bones to rub against each other during motion. This can eventually lead to a change in the shape of the joints, which may form bony growths, called bone spurs. Any joint can be affected, but DJD affects the feet, knees, hips, spine, and fingers more than any other joints. Painful and knobby bone growths in the fingers are also common. DJD often produces mild aching pain, but can become severe. Unlike many types of arthritis, DJD does not spread through the entire body, but usually concentrates in one joint where destruction occurs. Symptoms of DJD are pain in a joint during or after using it, discomfort in a joint before, during, or immediately after a change in the weather, swelling in joints, and bony lumps on the end or middle of the finger.

Rheumatoid Arthritis is a very painful, chronic inflammatory disease that is potentially disabling, characterized by inflammation of the joint lining. It is the second most common arthritis, which affects about 2.5 million Americans, mostly women. It can develop at any age, but usually strikes between the ages of 20 and 50. It is also a common type of arthritis among children, called juvenile rheumatoid arthritis. It can affect almost every joint in the body, but is most commonly seen in the hands. Unlike osteoarthritis, it can spread to different joints throughout the body, causing severe joint deformation. It is very difficult to control, making many of its victims less mobile and bedridden. Rheumatoid arthritis can cause weakness, fatigue, and loss of appetite, which can lead to weight loss and muscle pain.

Risk factors in developing rheumatoid arthritis are smoking, obesity, lack of exercise, stress, and an unhealthy diet.[27] Both rest and exercise are important in helping patients cope with the symptoms of rheumatoid arthritis. Rest helps fight fatigue and reduce joint inflammation. Exercise also preserves joint mobility and maintains joint flexibility in the body. People with rheumatoid arthritis have many emotional challenges as well as physical changes.

Gout is the third most common form of arthritis, affecting about one million people. Gout causes sudden severe attacks, usually in the big toe, called Podagra, but any joint can be affected. Gout is a metabolic disorder in which uric acid builds up in the blood and forms uric acid crystals in the joints. Gout can be related to kidney disease, medications, but it is usually related to diet.

There are many other forms of arthritis such as ankylosing spondylitis, psoriasis, systemic lupus erythematosus, fibromyalgia, and scleroderma. Many of the treatments for different forms of arthritis are the same. Osteoarthritis and rheumatoid arthritis are treated with medication such as Tylenol, aspirin, Aleve, Motrin-ib and corticosteroids. Surgery is recommended after long term destruction of a joint. Surgeons can realign a joint or replace the damaged joint with an artificial one. But the best way to prevent all forms of arthritis is to eat a majority of God's Original Diet and exercise on a regular basis.

Many patients are advised to lose weight and exercise when they are diagnosed with arthritis, because excess pounds put stress on weight bearing joints, especially the knees and hips. If a person already has arthritis in one knee and loses weight, it will reduce their chances of arthritis spreading to the other knee and may even relieve pain in the arthritic knee. Stress plays a role in arthritis as well. Stress in joints can worsen or even trigger certain types of arthritis, such as rheumatoid and osteoarthritis. Exercise plays a major role in controlling arthritis. Exercise such as swimming, walking, and stretching reduce joint pain and stiffness. Changing your diet and lifestyle can play the biggest role in preventing or defeating arthritis. Studies show that arthritis may come from a buildup of uric acid crystals. These crystals begin to penetrate the joints and bones of the body causing pain and immobility of the joints. The joints of the body are bathed in synovial fluid, which allows proper movement of bones around joints.

Uric acid crystals come from our diet, through eating excessive amounts of meat, dairy products, coffee, sodas, and processed unrefined foods.[28] When meats and other deadly food sit in the GI tract for long periods of time, they begin to secrete poisons, and uric acid is one of these poisons. Over time after continually eating excessive amounts of these dead foods, the body has to get rid of these uric acid crystals. The body has difficulty getting rid of dead foods in the GI tract that don't contain fiber, so the body decides to put the uric acid crystals in the muscles, bones, and joints. These uric acid crystals act like cement to the joints and bones causing joints to stiffen up, taking away joint motion and causing pain.

This is when we began to have symptoms of stiff and achy joints. As these crystals began to invade the joints and bones of the body, they begin to replace the synovial fluid, causing friction between the two opposing bones of the joint. This causes an autoimmune reaction in the body, causing destruction of the bones, joints, cartilage, and eventually leads to bone deformation. A buildup of uric acid crystals causes bones, joints, and muscles to absorb the crystals like a sponge. This is when we begin to suffer from rheumatoid and osteoarthritis, neuritis, sciatica, and other forms of arthritis.

If you grew up eating and drinking deadly foods such as meats, dairy products, fatty fried foods, coffee, teas, sodas, Kool-aid, sugary cereals, doughnuts, bagels, and other deadly foods, then about the time you turn 40, your diet may catch up with you in the form of arthritis.

These crystals can affect every joint in the body, from the ankles, knees, hips, spine, elbow, shoulder, all the way to the hand. Have you ever seen people with so many crystals in their joints that they cannot straighten out their back or close their hand? It is common in America, and we usually blame it on one thing; the fact that we are getting old. You are not getting old; your diet has finally caught up with you. Stop eating all those dead foods and you will see your health improve. There have been many people who have defeated arthritis simply by changing their diet. If you know someone who suffers from arthritis, do they eat lots of meats, dairy products, coffee, sodas, fried foods, refined processed foods, and other unhealthy foods? Probably so. Do they exercise on a regular basis? Probably not. Do they keep stress in their lives to a minimum? Probably not. Do they eat plenty of foods that grow from the earth? Probably not. Do they drink plenty of water? Probably not. If you want to prevent arthritis from invading your body, exercise on a regular basis, reduce stress in your life, and most importantly, "Eat the Way God Intended."

Diabetes

Diabetes comes from the Greek, meaning to pass a honey sweet liquid. Physicians as far back as the 17th century noted that diabetes was more commonly seen among the wealthy. At that time poor people lived mostly on farms and ate basic foods that grew from the earth. Only the wealthy could afford white flour and white sugar. During World War II the English government passed a law called the National Flour Act that prohibited the refining and processing of whole grain and sugar. During that period from 1941 to 1953, the diabetic mortality rate in England fell by 54%. The law was later rejected in 1953, and by 1955 the diabetic mortality rate was back up to pre-war levels. Diabetes is primarily seen in the Western world - the U.S. Canada, Australia, New Zealand, Sweden, and Europe. In China the incidence of diabetes is less than half that of the U.S., and yet, among Chinese people living in the U.S., the percentage of diabetes is the same as the U.S. population.

Diabetes is seen more in African Americans than any other race, but in Africa where the Western diet has not invaded, diabetes is not prevalent. It is estimated that worldwide about 100 million people have diabetes, and by 2010 this number will double. About 16 million people in the U.S. have some form of diabetes, and half don't know they are diabetic and have not yet been diagnosed.

The prevalence of diabetes is continuing to rise, as the U.S. population ages and more become obese. There are about 800,000 new cases of diabetes diagnosed each year, and about 194,000 deaths directly attributed to diabetes. Diabetes is the leading cause of adult blindness in the U.S., and it is the single leading cause of non-traumatic amputations and kidney failure. The most tragic thing about diabetes is that, many of the health problems associated with the condition can be prevented by maintaining a normal body weight, exercising, and eating the way God intended.

Diabetes is a group of conditions in which the body's sugar, glucose, levels in the blood are too high. When sugar levels get too high, the pancreas makes insulin which takes sugar and puts it inside the cells of the body to bring down the sugar level in the blood. Glucose is the main sugar that feeds the cells of the body, supplying them with energy, especially the brain. It is the nutrient that gives us energy to perform our daily activities. The pancreas is a gland near the stomach that secretes digestive enzymes and the hormone insulin. Under normal circumstances when we eat foods that contain proteins, fats, and carbohydrates, these nutrients are broken down into simpler, more easily absorbed sugars.

These nutrients are broken down into glucose, the most common sugar. Glucose is absorbed in the bloodstream and is used by body cells that need it for energy. When muscles or other tissues in the body need energy, they tell the pancreas to make insulin which in turn enters the bloodstream and attaches to glucose, and brings the glucose into the muscle cells for energy. If we eat a large meal and more sugar is absorbed through the bloodstream than the body needs at that time, the pancreas secretes insulin and the insulin puts the excess glucose into fat cells. This excess glucose stays in the fat cells until the body needs to use it. The body uses this backup supply of sugar when the fresh supply of sugar has run out. This backup sugar is usually needed in such activities as running, swimming, cycling, and other aerobic exercises because the body uses extra glucose for these exercises.

For example, if we eat a heavy breakfast in the mornings and run two hours later, our body will use the fresh supply of sugar that we ate for breakfast in the beginning of the run, but as we continue to run, the fresh supply of energy runs out and the body has to use the backup sugar which is stored in the fat cells to provide the energy necessary to continue to run. This is why exercising is helpful in losing weight, because it helps us use the backup sugar stored in fat cells. With diabetes the pancreas does not make enough insulin to bring glucose into cells for energy, or sometimes does not make any insulin at all. As diabetics continue to eat, glucose levels continue to rise in the blood without being taken to other tissues for energy. The glucose levels in the blood get so high, they spill into the urine and are passed out of the body unused. Over time this causes the body to lose important fuel that could have been used for energy, which leaves the patient very tired and starving for energy.

When this happens the body has to rely on protein and fat stored in the body to fuel itself for energy. As fat and protein begin to replace sugar in the bloodstream, it causes a shift in the blood's pH level, leaving it very acidic. In an acidic bloodstream, all the oxygen is not carried by red blood cells to cells throughout the body, eventually causing a diabetic coma, and even death. High sugar levels in the blood can also eventually cause damage to nerves, eyes, kidneys, heart, and blood vessels.

There are three types of diabetes - **insulin-dependent diabetes mellitus**, type 1 diabetes, non-insulin dependent diabetes mellitus, type 2 diabetes, and gestational diabetes, which occurs in women during pregnancy. Gestational diabetes usually ends after the baby is born, but is often a warning sign that if the woman doesn't change her lifestyle, she will eventually develop type 2 diabetes.

Insulin-Dependent Diabetes Mellitus (IDDM), also called type 1 diabetes, most often develops in children and young adults. For this reason type 1 diabetes was once called juvenile diabetes. In fact, it is one of the most common disorders found in children in the U.S. Each year between 11,000 and 12,000 children are diagnosed with type 1 diabetes. Type 1 diabetes can occur at any age, but usually appears between infancy and about 40 years of age, most typically in childhood or adolescence. Boys and girls are equally prone to type 1 diabetes. This condition can be inherited from a diabetic mother or father. Type 1 diabetes is less common but more severe than type 2 diabetes, and makes up about 5 to 10% of the diabetic population. In type 1 diabetes, cells in the pancreas that produce insulin are slowly destroyed, leading to insulin deficiency.

Without insulin to move glucose into the cells of the body, blood sugar levels become high, which is a condition known as hyperglycemia. When the body does not use the sugar, it spills into the urine and is eliminated. This leads to symptoms of weight loss, hunger, thirst, and weakness. These patients become dependent upon administered insulin in order to live normal lives. The exact cause of type 1 diabetes is not completely understood, but scientists believe many things can lead to this disease. Autoimmune responses in the body, viruses, and genetic abnormalities are all believed to be a cause of type 1 diabetes. Cow's milk is looked at as a cause of type 1 diabetes as well. A study found that a percentage of babies who are fed cow's milk go on to develop type 1 diabetes, and another study found that children fed cow's milk in the first eight days of life had twice the risk for developing type one diabetes than those on breast milk.[29]

Symptoms of type 1 diabetes include frequent urination, continuous bed wetting after toilet training, thirst for sweet and cold drinks, sudden weight loss, extreme hunger, weakness, blurred vision, changes in eyesight, and irritability. Children with type 1 diabetes may also have trouble learning and functioning in school.

Non-Insulin Dependent Diabetes Mellitus (NIDDM), also called type 2 diabetes, is the more common form of diabetes. It accounts for about 90% of adult diabetes. About 16 million Americans have type 2 diabetes and many are not even aware they have the disease. The difference between type 1 and type 2 diabetes is that the pancreas in type 2 diabetic patients produce variable and sometimes normal amounts of insulin, but they have abnormalities in the liver and muscle cells that resist the actions of insulin.

In a condition called insulin resistance, insulin tries to bring glucose into the cells of tissues, but the glucose cannot get inside the cells. Since the glucose cannot get into the cells of tissues for energy, it builds up in the bloodstream and spills into the urine. The body then has to use fat and protein in the body for energy, which can lead to a lack of oxygen in the blood due to fatty acid buildup.

Symptoms of type 2 diabetes include excessive thirst, increased urination, weakness, weight loss, and blurred vision. Fungal infections may occur under the breast or in the groin region. Women with type 2 diabetes may suffer with vaginal yeast infections and impotence may occur in men. Itching, severe gum disease, and unusual sensations, such as tingling and burning in the arms and legs can be signs of type 2 diabetes as well.

Hypoglycemia, low blood sugar, can occur in diabetics. When the pancreas makes too much insulin, it can take too much glucose out the bloodstream and cause a diabetic to go into shock. Symptoms of hypoglycemia are sweating, hunger, trembling, rapid heartbeat, confusion, weakness, disorientation, and, in worst cases, seizures, coma, and death. The major complications in both types of diabetes are due to blood vessel and nerve damage. Heart attacks account for about 60% and strokes account for about 25% of deaths in all diabetics. Both types of diabetes accelerate the progression of atherosclerosis, which may lead to coronary artery disease, heart attack, and stroke. In both types of diabetes, it is common for high blood pressure to develop, which can also lead to heart failure.

Nerve damage occurs in about 60 to 70% of diabetic patients, affecting sensation in the extremities. Symptoms include numbness, tingling, weakness, and burning sensations, starting in the fingers and toes moving up to the arms and legs. Nerve damage can become so bad that the diabetic patient cannot feel a blister, cut, scrapes, or other minor wounds on or in the skin. Neuropathy is worsened by vascular injury in diabetics, which can cause blood circulation problems in the legs and feet. With nerve and vascular damage, even a minor cut can cause deep tissue damage, causing an abnormally long time for the cut to heal. Because diabetics have extra glucose in the bloodstream, cuts and bruises are hard to heal, leaving bacteria too feed off the glucose.

Over time, if there is no blood supply to a particular area, it can cause gangrene, death of soft tissue, to set in that area of the body. In extreme cases of gangrene, the foot and leg have to be amputated because of a lack of blood and nerve supply to the area. Diabetes is responsible for more than half of all the lower limb amputations performed in the U.S. each year. Diabetes causes about 24,000 new cases of blindness a year, and is the leading cause of blindness in adults between the ages of 20 and 75. People with diabetes are also at higher risk for developing cataracts and certain types of glaucoma.

Obese type 2 diabetic women face a higher risk for uterine, breast, and endomentrial cancer. Diabetic women have early menopause, and pregnant diabetic women have a higher risk for birth defects.

Diabetes is diagnosed by the fasting plasma glucose test and the glucose tolerance test. Using the fasting plasma glucose test the patient fast for 8 hours, and then the glucose level in the blood is measured. If the blood sugar level is high after fasting for 8 hours, the patient is considered diabetic. This test is not always reliable. With the glucose tolerance test, patients are given a special glucose solution to drink, and blood sugar levels are measured two hours later. Normally, blood sugar levels increase after drinking the glucose solution, then return to normal after about two hours. In the diabetic, the blood sugar level starts out high and remains high.

Treatment for both types of diabetes is similar. Insulin is essential, and diabetics have to watch their diet. It is important for people with both types of diabetes to exercise. Many people have diabetes because of an unhealthy diet and lack of exercise. Exercise helps lower blood pressure and helps insulin take glucose into tissue cells for energy. Exercise also helps lower cholesterol levels in the blood, decrease body fat, and reduce the risk for heart disease. Studies show that people who engage in regular moderate exercise lower their risk for diabetes.[30] Brisk walking, running, cycling, and swimming are some of the best exercises for diabetes. Because glucose levels go up and down during exercise, people with diabetes should monitor their levels before, during, and after workouts.

Many diabetics are overweight which is usually what led to diabetes in the first place. Eating a healthy diet is the key to controlling diabetes, especially type 2. The recommendation for controlling diabetes is to eat a high fiber, low fat diet and limit salt intake. Diabetics are usually given drugs to help reduce weight and cholesterol levels and never told the right foods to eat. Diabetics are told to always carry hard sugary candy, sugary juices, white processed breads, or refined sugar packets, just in case their blood sugar gets low. Eating and drinking dead processed refined sugars will bring only temporary relief, but in the long run these dead foods complicate the diabetes even more. Diabetics should be taught about the quality of sugar. Sugar quality makes a big difference in the body, because the body prefers the sugars from fruits and vegetables - complex sugars - than from processed dead sugars. Simple sugars from processed foods cause dramatic rises in blood sugar, followed by dramatic drops in blood sugar. This is not healthy for anyone.

Complex sugars found in foods that grow from the earth, with the fibrous portions in tact, cause the blood sugar to rise very gradually, and then drop slowly too normal blood sugar levels. Refined sugars are missing many nutrients needed to control and prevent diabetes. Whole natural foods contain these valuable nutrients. Many doctors are starting to put diabetic patients on high protein diets that include heavy meats. A high protein diet controls the symptoms of diabetes better than a simple sugar diet, because it takes the body longer to breakdown proteins than it does to breakdown processed sugars. A high protein diet will not cause a constant rise and fall in blood sugar levels, but it will overload the GI tract, which leads to complications of heart disease, cancer, strokes, and kidney and liver disease.

Other factors that can contribute to diabetes are alcohol, dairy products, caffeine, and nicotine. You will never find diabetes in wild animals, yet household pets get diabetes frequently, because they eat like their owners.

If you are suffering from diabetes, start eating vegetables or whole fruits instead of sugary flavored juices. The majority of your diet should consist of vegetables because they contain less sugar. Exercise on a regular basis and reduce your stress. You will lose weight and prevent the damaging side effects of diabetes.

Osteoporosis

Osteoporosis involves loss of bone material. It is a condition that drains away the hardest substance in the body and happens slowly over a period of time, until one day a bone snaps or breaks unexpectedly. Osteoporosis is a very common condition, the 11th leading cause of death among women due to hip fractures. Osteoporosis is probably the most feared condition in postmenopausal women, and it leads to about 1.5 million fractures or breaks a year, often with complications. Men are also prone to osteoporosis, but it is seen mostly in women.

The simplest things in life can be very difficult for people who have osteoporosis. Stepping off a curb, hugging, and bending over to pick up something, can all cause bones fractures in people with osteoporosis. Osteoporosis is very simply, thinning of the bones. As it progresses, there is a gradual change of height, due to vertebras collapsing over time. It affects both the amount of bone tissue and the strength of bone tissue in the body. It is another disease that mostly affects the Western world - the U.S., England, Canada, and France - and is very rare in China, Africa, and Asia. It is common to lose bone in our youth, and when we do, our body normally replaces the old bone with new bone. Under normal conditions, each year somewhere between 10 to 30% of bones is being replaced, which mean it takes an average of about 5 years to turnover a complete set of bones. As we get older, this bone remolding gets slower, at about 21 years of age.

Unfortunately, bone breakdown doesn't slow down, and it may even accelerate as we get older. Gradual thinning of bone occurs with everyone over time, but in osteoporosis it is accelerated. At menopause, women begin to lose their bone mass about twice as fast as men, and after 5 to 6 years following menopause, women lose bone mass 6 times more quickly than men. Osteoporosis is detected by the use of a bone density test, called the single photon absorptiomentry, which shows if bone content has a tendency to fracture. This test measures how dense the bone is by using the forearm. It can also be used to check the density of the hip and spine.

X-rays should not be used to detect osteoporosis, because there must be a 35 to 40% calcium loss from the bone before it will show up on x-ray. By the time osteoporosis is seen on x-ray, it is too late to prevent it. The three major areas of bones where osteoporosis is found are the vertebra, wrist, and hip, especially the neck of the femur. The hip is the most serious of all bone fractures, and it can be disabling and life threatening, even leading to death. Osteoporosis is the leading cause of accidental death in older white women in the U.S. There are many risk factors for developing osteoporosis. Early menopause is a risk factor, especially if women have had a complete hysterectomy. The bone loss that follows menopause is due to loss of estrogen. Female ovaries begin to slow down the production of estrogen as early as the late 30's.

Ethnicity seems to play a factor in osteoporosis, because the lighter your complexion, the higher your risk for developing osteoporosis. This condition more heavily affects whites more than blacks.[31] Black women tend to have larger bones and more muscle mass than white women. With greater musculature, more pressure is put on the bone and that increases bone density.

What causes osteoporosis? Before I answer that, it is important to understand the function of bone. You may already know that bones provide a structure that holds us upright, and they respond to the pulling of muscles and gravity. Bones also repair themselves, meaning they are constantly making new bone. What you may not know is, that, besides protecting our internal organs and allowing us to move about, bones also store minerals. Important minerals such as calcium, phosphorus, magnesium, zinc, and other minerals are all stored in bones and taken out when the body needs them. When there is a low level of a particular mineral in the bloodstream, the body takes a fresh supply from bones. The same thing happens with osteoporosis.

We know that osteoporosis occurs because of a lack of calcium in the bones and teeth. Just like any other mineral, when the calcium in the bloodstream becomes low, the body goes into the bones to put more calcium into the bloodstream. Ninety nine percent of the body's calcium supply is stored in bone tissue and only 1% in the bloodstream. The calcium in the blood is much more important than the calcium in the bones, and it has a higher priority in the body than the other 99% of calcium in the bones. The 1% of calcium found in the bloodstream controls neuromuscular contractions, including the heartbeat, muscular relaxation, transmission of nerve impulses, clotting of blood, and other important functions. The 99% of calcium found in bones only helps maintain bone structure, meaning that the calcium in bones is not as important as the calcium in blood. So when calcium levels get low in the blood, the body will not hesitate to take calcium out of the bones to replace the calcium loss in blood. Therefore, it is important to eat plenty of foods containing quality calcium. Eating a lot of calcium alone does not prevent osteoporosis. Statistics show that countries with the highest calcium intake are the same countries with the most osteoporosis. Countries that have the lowest intake of calcium also have low incidence of osteoporosis.[32] It is the quality of calcium that plays a role in the development of osteoporosis. Many doctors tell their patients to get plenty of calcium, but doctors should teach their patients to get a good quality of calcium to prevent osteoporosis. The best calcium comes from foods that grow from the earth. What commercials and doctors don't focus on is the calcium to phosphorus ratio in the body. The average person takes in three to five times more phosphorus in their diet than they need. When we eat foods that contain lots of phosphorus, the body's bloodstream becomes acidic, so the body has to take calcium out of bone and put it into the bloodstrean to bring the pH level of the blood back to normal.

Remember, we are an alkaline species, meaning that the foods we eat should have an alkaline affect in the bloodstream, not an acidic effect. The pH of the bloodstream is very critical to our survival, therefore, whenever the pH level in the bloodstream shifts because of excess phosphorus, the body will not hesitate to remove calcium and other alkaline minerals from the bone, and put it in the blood to neutralize it. Every time we eat high protein meals, this reaction occurs in the body. This means that every time you eat and drink your meat, fatty foods, sodas, coffee, tea, cow's milk, and other dairy products, this reaction takes place, because all of these foods contain a high amount of phosphorus, which turns the bloodstream acidic.[33,34,35] If you eat these foods in excess, over a period of years, your body gradually takes too much calcium out your bones which eventually leads to osteoporosis. Smoking also leads to osteoporosis. In 1972, a study was done that showed that 94% of women with severe osteoporosis were smokers, and 88% of them had smoked more than a pack a day. When nicotine is absorbed in the blood, the blood becomes acidic, and calcium has to be taken out of bone to neutralize it.[36] Caffeine found in coffee, soda, tea, and other deadly drinks also cause an acidic effect in the bloodstream, which results in excessive amounts of calcium being taken out of bones. Alcohol has been shown to lead to osteoporosis, and the majority of cases of osteoporosis in men have occurred in male alcoholics, as early as in their 20's.[37] Antacids are associated with increasing the risk of osteoporosis. One reason is because they have a lot of aluminum in them. People who take large amounts of aluminum will also lose calcium from bones because aluminum increases calcium excretion. So, just because certain antacid commercials "say it has calcium, and it's what your body needs" does not mean your body is using the calcium. Antacids, even though they contain calcium, actually decrease calcium absorption because they neutralize stomach acid.[38]

We are told to drink plenty of cow's milk, yogurt, and eat lots of dairy products, because it has plenty of calcium. It is true that cows' milk has plenty of calcium, but it has more phosphorus and fat than calcium. Therefore, cow's milk causes an acidic reaction in the bloodstream and the body has to take calcium out of bone to neutralize the blood. Cow's milk and other dairy products don't prevent osteoporosis, they cause it.[39]

We are also told to eat and drink sugary-flavored fruit juice and cereals that have added calcium. You cannot compare the calcium in man-made foods to the calcium in God's foods. If you want to prevent osteoporosis, you should eat plenty of vegetables. All vegetables and raw nuts are good sources of calcium. Other great sources of calcium are pineapples and oranges.

Weight-bearing exercises also help prevent osteoporosis. Exercising on a regular basis - walking, biking and running - helps to build and maintain strong bones.[40] Physical fitness reduces the risk of fracture in older people, because of better balance, muscle strength, and agility, which makes them less likely to fall. But don't run for long periods of time everyday, because it has a negative impact on your bones. Running for long periods of time without stopping can cause osteoporosis, because bones don't have adequate time to replace old bone cells with new bone cells. Remember, rest is good.

If you want to prevent osteoporosis, avoid excessive amounts of meat, fast foods, dairy products, alcohol, coffee, sodas, tea, cigarettes, and cigars. Keep your stress level to a minimum. Get plenty of sunlight because the sun's rays allow the body to produce vitamin D, which helps put calcium in bones.[41] Eat plenty of fruits and vegetables that grow from the earth, because these foods have the best source of calcium.

Fibroids

Uterine fibroids are benign (non-cancerous) tumors that are made of the smooth muscles of the uterus. They are found in the wall of the uterus and may even appear on the cervix. They can range in size from as small as a pea, to as large as a watermelon. Fibroids develop most commonly in women who are in their thirties and forties, but they can develop much earlier and later. About 30% of all women over 35 years of age will develop fibroids. Fibroids are usually grayish to white in color and are round, firm, and ring-shaped. Once fibroids develop they may return, even if they are surgically removed.

Fibroids cause lower abdominal or back pain and they can cause urinary problems. If fibroids press against the ureters, the tubes that carry urine from the kidneys to the bladder, they block the flow of urine, which may lead to kidney damage. Fibroids can also put pressure on the rectum and cause constipation.[42]

Fibroids cause heavier menstruation, which could lead to anemia. Extremely large fibroids can interfere with a pregnancy, or may even cause infertility, because they take up too much space in the uterus.[43] Fibroids can also block the fallopian tubes, meaning that after leaving the ovaries, a woman's eggs will be blocked from entering the uterus, preventing fertilization.

Other symptoms of fibroids are a tender and achy feeling of labor-like pains, pressure in the lower legs, painful sexual intercourse, incontinence and repeated urinary tract infections.[44] Chances of getting fibroids are higher in women who have not been pregnant and women who have a family history of fibroids. African American women get fibroids more than any other, although women who live in Africa don't appear to have as high an incidence of fibroids.[45] All women are at risk for fibroids during phases of their lives when estrogen levels are high. A high fatty diet can greatly increase estrogen levels in the body.[46] Fibroids usually start to grow right after puberty, although they are not usually detected until a woman reaches young adulthood. Other risk factors for fibroids is the age a young girls starts to menstruate because the younger you start menstruation, the longer your body will be exposed to estrogen.

Treatment for fibroids include watchful waiting, which is waiting to see if the tumor is growing and spreading across the uterus. In most cases the doctor never tells the patient about her diet while they are in this phase. They are usually given iron supplements to help prevent anemia, and told to come back if the tumor gets any bigger. If the women are about to go into menopause, they are told to wait, because tumors usually shrink after menopause, due to a lack of estrogen production. Women may be given aspirin, Advil, Motrin, or other drugs to help with menstrual pain. When non-surgical procedures don't work, the standard operation for removing fibroids is a total hysterectomy, removal of the uterus and cervix, and sometimes the ovaries. It is very common for a woman with fibroids to be scared into having a hysterectomy. Fibroids are the most common reason for hysterectomies in the U.S., accounting for about 30% of all hysterectomies performed in the country - about 200,000 a year. Studies now show that about 50% of all hysterectomies performed in general, may have been clearly unnecessary, while about 20% of them could have been avoided by using alternative approaches.

Fibroids don't just happen to appear in the body, something has to cause these fats to form on or in the uterus. Eating excessive amounts of saturated fats from animals, margarine, dairy products, and fried foods will cause the body to deposit these fats in the uterus and other organs.[47] Smoking, alcohol, coffee, sodas, and other caffeine foods also cause fibroid formation.[48] The best way to reduce your chance of developing fibroids is to eat a majority of foods that grow from the earth. Fruits and vegetables don't cause tumor formation, they prevent it.

Another great way to prevent fibroids is to exercise on a regular basis. Exercise reduces fat in the body, which reduces the estrogen levels in the body. Walking, running, cycling, and swimming are great exercises that help reduce fibroids.[49] These exercises help you sweat and release toxins and other waste from of the body. Reduce your stress, and most importantly, eat a majority of God's Original Diet.

Asthma and Allergies

Asthma and allergies are chronic illnesses caused by inflammation of the lungs. When the lungs are inflamed, the airways become constricted and filled with fluid, which leads to shortness of breath, coughing, and wheezing. Symptoms of **asthma** include a persistent dry cough, coughing during the night that disturbs sleep, wheezing, and shortness of breath. Asthma is a struggle for breath, and people who suffer from it constantly struggle for breath. It affects 4.1 million children under the age of 18, and is the leading serious chronic illness among children.

Asthma causes the normal functions designed to protect the lungs from harmful material to function abnormally. When the muscles of the lungs come into contact with foreign matter, the normal reaction is to cough or sneeze it out of our bodies, but with asthma, the muscles in the lungs contract more than normal and tighten. The tightening of the muscles then causes the mucus membranes in the lungs to swell, which reduces the diameter of the airways, making it very difficult to breathe. There are many things that can trigger an asthma attack, such as stress, cold temperature, a change in weather, pollen, dust, pets, cigarette smoke, aerosol sprays, etc. Asthma can affect people of any race, age, or sex, but there are some people who are more prone to this disease.

Studies show that children of smokers are twice as likely to develop asthma as the children of non-smokers.[50] Studies show that healthy babies born to women who smoked during pregnancy, have abnormally narrow airways, which can cause them to suffer from asthma later in life. This can lead to weakness of the lungs in children making them more prone to chronic lung disease in the future. African Americans have a higher rate of asthma than any other race.

Asthma is treated with many drugs, such as bronchodialators, corticosteroids, and allergy injections. To avoid asthma it is important to build up your immune system. The stronger your immune system, the better your body will be able to fight off allergies, dust, pollen, and other materials that make your lungs go into spasm. The best way to build up your immune system is to eat foods that grow from the earth. Fruits and vegetables do not destroy the immune system, because they build it up. The only foods that break your immune system down are man-made foods. Excessive amounts of meats, dairy products, fried foods, smoking, coffee, tea, alcohol, and sodas will only break down your immune system.

Allergies are believed to play a role in almost all diseases. The body naturally has the ability to distinguish self from non-self, between the internal world and the external world. Self is matter that is naturally found in the body, and non-self is matter that is not naturally found in the body, such as pollen, dust, fumes from aerosol sprays, etc. An allergy is a sensitive reaction in the body that occurs in a hypersensitive state after re-exposure to an allergen. The body recognizes the allergen as not being a part of the body, non-self, and tries to get rid of it as soon as possible. As the body gets rid of the allergen, the person experiences an allergic reaction. The areas where we are most likely to show symptoms of allergies are the lungs, GI tract, skin, and musculoskeletal system. All allergic conditions are tied to the immune system.

Allergies are originally developed as early as a baby's development in utero. Although the baby does not have much protection in the mother's womb, there are things from the outside world that can effect their development of allergies. If a mother constantly eats the same foods while pregnant, the child can develop an allergy to that particular food. While a mother is pregnant the immune system begins to develop antibodies to every antigen that the mother has encountered. The better the baby is protected while in utero, the less likely the baby will develop allergies later in life.

When a baby is born, its immune system is very immature, and the GI tract is weak as well. The size of a baby's stomach at birth is about the size of a chicken egg, which means that it cannot hold very much. Secretory IgA is an antibody, which lines the digestive and respiratory tracts and protects the body against invading organisms. It is found in adults and little is found in babies. Since babies have very little Secretory IgA, they are easily infected, especially if the mother does not breast-feed. Unfortunately, most mothers don't breast-feed, and they give the baby solid foods before they grow teeth to chew food. This is one of the worst things you can do to your child because it is the origin of a lot of digestive problems and allergies that last a lifetime.

Most of the time we feed babies cereal when they don't have enough salivary amylase, the enzyme necessary to breakdown starches, to digest cereals and milk, which causes the baby to develop colic. This usually sets the foundation for all kinds of health problems later in life. The most common food allergen is cow's milk. Many studies have proven that introducing your baby to cow's milk contributes to allergies and asthma.[51] In fact, most allergies would be nonexistent if humans did not drink cow's milk.

Earth-grown foods help build up the immune system, making it tolerate foreign matter better. It is also important that we don't eat food, that is not good for the immune system. Common foods that cause allergic reactions are eggs, cow's milk, chocolate, shellfish, and sugary, refined citrus fruit.[52] Most of these foods are high in protein and fat, and when given to infants, it may start a pre-stage for many allergies.

The reason citrus fruits are a common allergen is because we drink too much of it.

When we eat or drink foods everyday we eventually become allergic to it. Let's take orange juice, for example, because there are many people who are allergic to orange juice. These people probably used to drink orange juice everyday and probably drank between 2 to 3 cups a day. This is why nature made oranges and not orange juice. Drinking two to three cups of orange juice a day is like eating 8 to 10 oranges, and we cannot eat that many oranges a day. Another reason that citrus juices cause allergies is because they are not pure freshly squeezed fruit juices. Freshly squeezed orange juice very seldom produces allergens.

Most people who have allergies as children don't really outgrow them, and in many cases, the body converts the symptoms as we grow older. For example, the child who has hay fever as a child may have colitis, arthritis, or migraines as adults, if they don't change their lifestyle. If you want to prevent asthma and allergies, eat foods that help build up the immune system. To prevent asthma and many allergies, don't give babies solid foods until they have grown enough teeth to chew with.

Another way to prevent allergens is to breast-feed because it contains immunities which fight against allergens. Breast-feeding can reduce autoimmune diseases from developing later in life.[53] Exercising on a regular basis will improve the strength of the lungs and airways, making them less sensitive to asthma and allergies.[54] Exercises such as walking, running, swimming, and cycling are great exercises to strengthen the lungs. Eating healthy foods and exercising on a regular basis will greatly improve your fight against asthma and allergies. This helps to build up the immune system, allowing the body to fight off foreign matter without causing an allergic reaction.

The Common Cold

Everyone gets a cold at some point in their life. It is the most common illness that people suffer from today. On average, Americans develop two to four colds a year, which totals about 200 million colds a year. Colds are most prevalent among children, and seem to be related to their lack of resistance to infection, and their contacts with other children in schools and daycare centers.

It is very important to feed our children foods that will help build up their immune system, so that they will be able to fight off viruses, such as the common cold. It is estimated that children have six to ten colds a year, and for children in school the number can be as high as 12 colds a year. These numbers decrease as the child ages and their immune system becomes stronger. The economic impact of the common cold is very high. It is estimated that about 66 million cases of colds each year require medical attention, or result in restricted activity.

There are over 200 different viruses that are known to cause the symptoms of the common cold. The most common form of the common cold is the rhinovirus. The rhinovirus seldom produces severe illness, but does cause the common symptoms of fatigue, runny nose, coughing, and sneezing. Other viruses, such as the flu virus, can cause infections and respiratory infections.

In the United States, most colds occur around the fall and winter. Many people feel that cold weather causes colds, but evidence has not shown this to be true. The cold epidemic starts each year in late August and the incidence of colds increases slowly for a few weeks and remains high until April.

Most cold-causing viruses survive better in low humidity, and the humidity is much lower in the winter and fall months. Cold weather also makes the lining of the nasal passages drier, which can makes us more vulnerable to viral infection. Symptoms of the common cold usually begin two to three days after the infection. These symptoms often include nasal discharge, swelling of the sinus membranes, coughing, sneezing, sore throat, difficulty breathing, and headaches. Fevers occur with colds, to heat the body to a certain temperature in order to kill the virus. Cold symptoms can last from 2 to 14 days, depending on how strong your immune systems is, with the average cold lasting about a week. Cold viruses cause infections by suppressing the body's immune system.

The immune system is the body's defense system, which fights off viruses, bacteria, and other foreign matter that our body comes into contact with on a day-to-day basis. The body's first line of defense is mucus, produced by the membranes in the nose and throat. When we breathe in foreign matter - pollen, dust, bacteria, viruses, and other matter - mucus traps the material. As a defense mechanism, we cough or sneeze to get rid of the matter. Sometimes a virus, such as the cold virus, is able to penetrate the mucus membrane and enter a cell, the cell then starts to make other viruses, just like the cold virus. As more and more cold viruses are made, they begin to attack normal surrounding cells, breaking down the body. This is when we begin to have symptoms of the cold. When the body's immune system realizes it is under attack, it sends special blood cells, called white blood cells, to kill the cold virus. While white blood cells are fighting against cold viruses, we have symptoms of tiredness, drowsiness, lack of appetite, and we just want to stay in the bed.

Colds are spread in various ways, but the most common way is by touching infectious viruses on the skin and on environmental surfaces and then touching the eyes or the nose. The second way is by inhaling cold viruses that are transported in the air. The cold can be easily transmitted to another person about the fourth day after infection, when the virus is at its peak in the nasal passages. People who are more likely to get colds are people who smoke or are around a person that smokes. The risk of a cold is increased by exposure to cigarette smoke, because smoke can injure the lung's airways and damage the cilia, tiny hair-like filaments that keep the airways clear.

People who inhale toxic fumes, industrial smoke, and other air pollutants are also at risk for colds. Stress also increases a person's susceptibility to a cold because stress decreases the function in every system in the body, therefore making the body more susceptible to viruses and other diseases. The most important factor that contributes to colds is diet - people don't eat foods that build up their immune system to help them fight colds. The simplest and most effective way to prevent colds is to wash your hands. Avoid touching your eyes or nose to prevent cold virus from entering your body. Common medical treatments for the cold are to drink plenty of fluids, and take aspirin or Tylenol to relieve a headache or fever.

Colds are a way for the body to get rid of excess mucus. When you have eaten a certain amount of mucus-forming foods, and the body has stored them in various areas, there comes a time when the body has to get rid of it. There are a variety of ways that the body gets rid of mucus that has accumulated in the body, but the most common way is through a cold. If you eat excessive amounts of mucus-forming foods like refined sugars, cakes, pies, dairy products (eggs, butter, cheese, milk), and white processed breads, over time they begin to form mucus in the body and the body has to eventually get rid of it.

If you eat yogurt, white breads, white rice, bagels and other refined processed foods, these foods will eventually lead to colds because of the mucus they form.[55] And we cannot forget the main cause of colds in kids, which is cow's milk. Cow's milk causes mucus to form in the body, especially in infants, and can lead to ear infections, colds, flu, colic, and similar illnesses.[56]

When the body feels that it has too much mucus, it gets rid of it by cleaning itself. If you cut down on the mucus-forming foods that you eat, you will have fewer colds, bronchitis, and flu. If you start eating more life-giving foods, you will have fewer colds.

As a young lad, I would catch colds about four times a year. I had cow's milk everyday with my cereals, because just like many other families, my mom thought cow's milk did a body good. I suffered with mucus everyday in the form of colds or sinus problems. I had yearly sinus infections, and I blew my nose constantly, probably around 50 times a day. I could blow mucus, or we used to call it 'snot', out of my nose up to twenty yards.

My head was constantly clogged with mucus and sometimes I could blow my nose so hard that mucus would come out my eyeball socket. I remember my mom giving me chicken soup, cough drops, and lemon juice mixed with eggs and honey, thinking that it would speed up the body's process of getting rid of the cold, when, in fact, all these remedies did was slow down my body's process of getting rid of the cold. Now that I have changed my diet and eliminated mucus-forming foods, I don't suffer from sinus problems as I did when I was a child. Now that I have eliminated cow's milk, ice cream, eggs, Kool-aid, and other mucus-forming foods, I don't suffer from colds four times a year.

If you are tired of suffering from colds, stop eating mucus-forming foods, exercise on a regular basis, and keep stress to a minimum, but most importantly, eat the way God intended.

Multiple Sclerosis

Multiple Sclerosis or MS is a disease that affects the brain and spinal cord. It was first diagnosed in 1849, but its earliest known symptoms date back to the fourteenth century. MS can be disabling, but the vast majority of patients are mildly affected. It is an autoimmune disease that damages the myelin sheaths of the nerve cells. The myelin sheath is a fatty insulation, which covers nerve fibers, and its function is to provide communication between the brain and spinal cord through electrical impulses. In MS this communication is interrupted. MS means that there is hardening of the nerves in multiple areas of the spinal cord or brain, similar to arteriosclerosis where the arteries become hard.

For example, when you touch a hot stove, messages from your hand go to your brain, telling the brain that your hand is on something hot. Your brain then interprets this information and sends a message to the hand allowing you to pull your hand off the hot stove. This process happens so quickly that the exact time cannot be measured, it can only be estimated. These messages or electrical impulses go through the myelin sheath of the nerves. When our nerves become hardened, as in MS, these messages are not received in various areas of the body, depending on where the sclerosis or hardening has taken place. MS is not fatal, but a patient with MS has a life expectancy that is, on average, six years shorter than normal. MS, just like most other diseases, is mostly seen in the Western World - the U.S. Canada, and Europe. MS is extremely rare in countries such as Asia and Africa, where the majority of foods eaten, grow from the earth. However MS is found in African Americans and Asians who have adopted the traditional American diet.

Patients diagnosed with MS may be told that the disease is life-long and that symptoms will only get worse. It is estimated that the annual costs of MS in the U.S. is more than 2.5 billion dollars. Symptoms of MS vary greatly among each patient. Most commonly, MS first manifests itself as a series of attacks, followed by a complete or partial remission phase as symptoms mysteriously lesson and sometimes disappear, only to return later after a period of stability. The initial symptom of MS is often blurred or double vision with red-green distortion or even blindness in one eye. Many MS patients experience muscle weakness in the arms and legs and difficulty with coordination and balance. These symptoms may be severe enough to impair walking or standing. In the worst cases of MS, partial or complete paralysis may occur. Other MS patients experience abnormal sensory feelings such as numbness, prickling, uncontrollable tremors, impaired speech, dizziness, and hearing loss. Bowel and bladder dysfunction may also occur in about 75% of MS patients.[57]

Treatments for MS are corticosteriods, to reduce the inflammation of the brain and spinal cord, and interfons to suppress the immune response.

Studies do show that people who eat diets low in fat have a much lower risk for developing MS. MS is most often seen in people who eat the standard American diet. Studies done on people who have died with or from MS, have shown that their brain tissues contained a higher amount of saturated fat than people who did not have the disease. This means that your diet may play a role in the development of MS. Other studies have found that kids who are fed cow's milk grow up with a greater chance of developing MS, than children who are fed mother's breast milk.[58]

Researchers have found that a nutrient called linoleic acid helps make up the myelin sheath found in the nervous system. Linoleic acid is a polyunsaturated fatty acid believed to be helpful in preventing MS. Linoleic acid is an essential nutrient needed for the development of the nervous system, which is where MS attacks. Cow's milk contains about one-fifth the amount of lenoleic acid that is found in mother's milk, which means when you feed your infant formula made from cow's milk or just plain cow's milk, you may be depriving them from developing a healthy nervous system, which may lead to MS in the future.[59]

Mother's milk contains the necessary amount of linoleic acid for infants to develop a healthy and functional nervous system. Linoleic acid is also found in the oils of nuts and seeds, such as safflower and sunflower oils, and in rye, wheat, germ, corn, soybean, oats, peanuts, Brazil nuts, and sesame oil. A healthy diet of fruits and vegetables helps control the function of the nervous system, and the normal transmission of nerve impulses.

Magnesium is a vital mineral used for the conduction of nerve impulses and muscle contraction. Potassium helps in the transmission of impulses along nerve fibers. Vitamins help build up and protect the nervous system. The B vitamins are essential in maintaining proper nerve function. Thiamine (B1), Niacin (B2), and Cobalmine (B12) all help the growth and development of the neuron cell, and the synthesis or making of the myelin sheath. Other antioxidant vitamins, mainly vitamins A, C, and E, help protect the nervous system from a variety of degenerative changes involving the cells and fibers of the nerves. These antioxidants also help protect the myelin sheath of the nervous system from degenerative changes. Antioxidants protect the nervous system by converting damaging free radicals into harmless matter, which is excreted out the body. All of these great minerals are prevalent in foods that grow from the earth. Magnesium is found in green leafy vegetables, fresh legumes, nuts and whole grains.

Potassium is prevalent in fruits and vegetables, and all the vitamins that your body needs to function properly are found abundantly in fruits and vegetables. This means that your diet may play a big role in developing MS, because there are essential nutrients from foods that your body needs for the nervous system to function properly. If the body does not get these particular nutrients, the nervous system may develop problems, including diseases like MS. The standard American diet, which consists of cow's milk and high animal fat, provides a good environment for producing MS.

Another disease called Parkinson's, which is similar to MS, may also be due to diet. Parkinson's disease is developed because of a loss of brain cells that produce a chemical called dopamine. Dopamine is important in the function of muscle activity. It is recommended that patients suffering with Parkinson's take plenty vitamin B6 (pyridoxine) because it is necessary in the production and metabolism of dopamine. Vitamin B6 and other B vitamins, which play important roles in the development of the brain and spinal cord, are found in earth-grown foods. If you want to prevent these diseases, exercise on a regular basis, keep stress to a minimum, and eat plenty of fruits and vegetables.

Kidney Failure

Kidney Failure is usually due to diabetes or high blood pressure.[60] Your kidneys are two bean-shaped organs that are about the size of your fist. Their job is to filter waste by-products that accumulate in the blood after the digestion of food. They are located near the middle of your back, just below the rib cage. Everyday the kidneys process about 200 quarts of blood and separate about 2 quarts of waste products from the blood. This waste becomes urine, which flows to your urinary bladder where it is stored, until enough urine builds up in the bladder for urination.

In addition to the kidneys removing waste, they also stimulate the making of red blood cells. The kidneys also help regulate blood pressure and help the bones maintain an adequate amount of calcium.

Symptoms of kidney disease are frequent headaches, fatigue, nausea, vomiting, and loss of appetite. Some people's hands and feet swell due to fluid buildup.

I like to compare the kidneys to the oil filters in a car. An oil filter filters out dirt, grease, and other particles in motor oil to keep the car engine clean. The kidneys filter out waste in the bloodstream to keep the blood clean. Just like oil is the life blood of a car, blood is the life of the body, and the filters play an important role in keeping motor oil and blood clean.

When we put low quality foods in our bodies for long periods of time, our kidneys will eventually stop functioning and breakdown. Some of us take better care of our vehicles than we do our own bodies. I have seen people who love to smoke, but would not smoke in their vehicles.

Treatment for kidney failure is either dialysis or a kidney transplant. Left untreated, kidney failure will lead to coma, seizures, and eventually death. Dialysis involves sending blood through a machine that filters out waste products and then returning clean blood to the body to carry out its normal function. A transplanted kidney is usually placed close to the urinary bladder and functions as a normal kidney.

These procedures can be prevented if we live a healthy life and eat healthy foods. Man-made foods are dangerous to the kidneys. When we eat excessive amounts of man-made foods, we are not providing our body with the best fuels. Excessive amounts of protein and fat from animals will eventually lead to high blood pressure and cause the kidneys to breakdown.[61] Cholesterol speeds up kidney failure by building up on the inside walls of your blood vessels, causing the heart to pump blood harder through the blood vessels in the kidneys. Remember, excess cholesterol comes into the body through diet. Salt raises blood pressure, which also causes the heart to pump blood harder through blood vessels in the kidneys. This excessive hard pumping by the heart can eventually lead to kidney failure. Nicotine and caffeine, like salt, also raise the blood pressure, eventually causing kidney failure.

Animals in the wild don't suffer from kidney failure, because they eat the foods that

God intended for them to eat. Fruits and vegetables don't damage the kidneys. If you want strong kidneys, eat a majority of earth-grown foods, and keep stress to a minimum.

Kidney and Gallstones

Kidney stones are one of the most common disorders of the urinary tract and more than one million cases of kidney stones are diagnosed each year. It is estimated that 10% of all people will have a kidney stone at some point in their lives. A kidney stone develops from crystals that separate from urine and build up in the inner surfaces of the kidney. They may contain various combinations of chemicals, but almost all types of kidney stones contain high amounts of calcium.

Two of the most common kidney stones are calcium oxalate and calcium phosphate. Calcium is part of a person's normal diet, and makes up important parts of the body such as bones and muscles. Kidney stones strike most people between 30 and 40 years of age, and once a person has more than one stone, he or she is more likely to develop others.[62] Usually the first symptom of a kidney stone is extreme pain. When a stone moves in the urinary tract, causing irritation or blockage, it causes sudden pain.

Usually, a person feels a sharp, cramping pain in the back and side, in the area of the kidney, or in the lower abdominal. Sometimes nausea, vomiting, chills, and fever occur with kidney pain. If the stone is too large to pass, the pain continues as the muscles try to squeeze the stone along into the bladder. As the stone grows and moves, it can scrape the muscles of the urinary tract, causing blood in the urine. Treatment for kidney stones is surgery to remove the stones.

Gallstones are formed from bile, a fluid composed of salts, cholesterol, and other chemicals. About 75% of the gallstones found in the U.S. population are formed from cholesterol.

Cholesterol only makes up about five percent of bile, and it must be properly balanced with other bile salts. If too much cholesterol is secreted by the liver into the bile, gallstones may form. That means the more cholesterol in the diet, the higher the chance for developing gallstones. Gallstones are very common, but only about 10% of people with gallstones actually become symptomatic. Symptoms of gallstones are indigestion, fever, vomiting, nausea, and pain when breathing. More severe symptoms of gallstones are rapid heartbeat and a drop in blood pressure. A person will normally remain asymptomatic, unless a stone blocks the gallbladder duct.

People who most commonly have gallstones are the 4 F's - fat, fertile, forty, and female. Gallstones are more likely to develop in men and women who are overweight, and who consume a diet high in cholesterol, saturated fats, and refined sugars. Every year about 500,000 people have their gallbladders removed. Surgical removal of the gallbladder is one of the most common surgical procedures performed on women.

If you want to prevent kidney stones and gallstones, eat a majority of foods that grow from the earth. Kidney stones are made mostly of calcium and gallstones are made mostly of cholesterol. When we eat excessive amounts of meats, and fatty foods, remember, the body has to take calcium out of bone to maintain the blood pH level and to help breakdown the proteins in meat. This excess calcium, and the calcium we are getting through our diet from drinking cow's milk, and other dairy products, spills over into the urine causing the formation of kidney stones. The body cannot use this excess calcium and it doesn't have time to get rid of it, because we are constantly eating dead foods. So the body puts the excess calcium in the blood, which eventually leads to the formation of kidney stones.[62]

When we reduce or eliminate dead foods from our diet, we prevent the formation of stones. Foods that are in God's Original Diet do not cause the formation of stones.

Cavities

Cavities begin as holes that form in teeth, eventually leading to tooth decay. It is very important to take care of your teeth, so that we can continue to eat and enjoy foods. We have been told that if we brush our teeth after every meal, we reduce our chances of having cavities. This may be true, to a certain extent, but most toothpaste serves only one purpose, they make our breath smell a little fresher.

Cavities are to teeth, as osteoporosis is to bone. Just like in bones, calcium is stored in the teeth. Calcium helps keep teeth hard for chewing foods, but when we start to eat and drink unhealthy foods, eventually cavities start to form, leading to tooth loss. When calcium is taken out of teeth, toothaches, cavities, and tooth decay will eventually form in the mouth. The same foods that cause osteoporosis will cause tooth decay, especially sugary foods. Most of the patients that dentist see in their office are there because of their diets. I am sure that many dentists don't inform their patients that their diets cause the majority of their tooth problems, because they simply don't know. Filling in cavities does not get to the primary cause of why cavities form in the first place.

Most of our children only drink sodas, Kool-aid, sugary-flavored fruit drinks, and eat candy, sugar-coated cereals, cakes, and pies, and when cavities form in their mouth, parents wonder why. The best way to prevent cavities from developing is to eat foods from the earth. The sugar in oranges, apples, pineapples, sugarcane, watermelon, and other fruits don't cause tooth decay, they help prevent it. Vegetables don't cause tooth decay, they prevent cavities. Raw nuts and seeds don't take calcium out of teeth and cause cavities; they provide the body with a good source of calcium. The second best way to prevent cavities is to floss your teeth after meals. This helps to remove food that has accumulated between the gums and teeth.

Cavities come from the foods that we eat. If all we eat and drink are excessive amounts of meats, sodas, teas, Kool-aid, coffee, hard candy, candy bars, sugar coated cereals, cakes and cookies, don't be surprised if cavities form in your mouth.[64] To prevent cavities, eat a majority of earth grown foods.

Headaches

Headaches are very common and many people suffer with them everyday. Headaches can be a symptom of many different problems. Common types of headaches include tension, migraine, cluster, and sinus headaches and it is common for people to feel a combination of all these headaches at one time. Headache pain occurs in the tissues covering the brain and in the muscles and blood vessels around the scalp, neck, and face. Common causes of headaches are stress, anxiety, lack of sleep, and diet.

Tension headaches, also called stress and muscular headaches, are often experienced in the forehead or the back of the head and neck and sometimes in both regions. They are described as a tightness of the scalp or neck and soreness in the shoulders. They can last from minutes to days at a time, and may even occur daily. Many people who suffer from tension headaches are under lots of stress, and many are depressed.

There are two different types of migraine headaches - common or classic migraines. Both are about the same, with the only difference being that classic migraine sufferers have a warning sign that the headache is about to occur.

Common migraines account for 80% of all migraines. Sufferers of common migraine may have symptoms of nausea, vomiting, cold hands, tremor, dizziness, and sensitivity to light and sound. Some warning signs that classic migraines, are about to occur are visual disturbances, smelling of strange odors, speech disturbances, pain in and behind the eyes, and numbness in the arms or legs. A typical migraine headache produces throbbing pain on one side of the head, often accompanied by nausea and vomiting. If untreated, attacks usually last from 4 hours to 3 days.

After a migraine attack, there is usually a phase in which the patient may feel exhausted, and mentally confused for a while. Almost half the women who experience migraines, usually experience them while they are on their menstrual cycles. Common factors that contribute to migraines are foods that can cause allergic reactions, such as cheese, cow's milk, chocolate, salt, artificial sweeteners, nitrates, barbecue, and smoked meats. Smoking, alcohol, hormones and birth control pills have also been known to cause migraines.[66]

Cluster headaches cause severe stabbing pain centered in one eye. People often awaken with them a few hours after they go to bed. Associated symptoms include excessive tearing, drooping eyelid, and a stuffy or runny nose, which all occur on the same side as the pain. Patients suffering from cluster headaches have a tendency to become restless, whereas migraine patients have a tendency to sleep. People who suffer from cluster headaches may pace the floor, or even bang their heads against walls and doors in an attempt to cope with or relieve the pain. Attacks last about 30 to 90 minutes, although they can last as long as three hours. Attacks occur for 4 to 8 weeks then disappear for about 18 months, with headache-free periods in between. During the active period sufferers can experience one or more bouts a day, or as few as one every other day. Ninety percent of all cluster patients are male, most between the ages of 20 to 30. Cluster headaches are usually associated with stress, excessive smoking, and excessive alcohol intake.[67]

Sinus headaches usually occur around the eye, across the checks, or over the forehead. They are usually mild in the mornings and increase in severity as the day progresses. Sinus headaches are usually due to infection, usually with fever, due to blockage of sinus ducts, which prevents normal drainage. Symptoms of sinus headaches are fever, runny nose, congestion, and sinus infections. To avoid sinus headaches you should avoid eating mucus-forming foods as much as possible.

There are many other causes of headaches such as high blood pressure, tumors, caffeine, hunger, and fevers. Most headaches can be prevented, if you eat the way God intended.

Most headaches come from eating man made foods, which put major stress on the arteries and muscles of the body. Foods such as cow's milk, cheeses, chocolate, cigarettes, alcohol, smoked meats, coffee, and sodas will all eventually lead to the suffering of headaches. These foods should never be eaten, and will only lead to sickness and disease.

Foods that grow from the earth do not put stress on the body. Eating fruits and vegetables help you control your stress better. Eating raw nuts and seeds helps your body fight against headaches, not cause them. If you want to decrease or prevent headaches, reduce your stress, exercise on a regular basis, and eat a majority of God's Original Diet.

Impotence

Impotence, also called erectile dysfunction, is becoming more common among males. A few years ago, this was a subject that most males did not talk about, because they were ashamed. If peers knew that you were impotent, you would probably become the topic of many jokes, but impotence is no joking matter. It affects many people, young and old, rich and poor. Males are starting to talk more about this issue as more of them begin to find out that they are not alone. Impotence is the consistent inability to sustain an erection sufficient for sexual intercourse. It can be described as a total inability to achieve erection, or it can be where a male can sustain erection for a brief period, but not long enough to have sexual intercourse.

It is estimated that impotence effects 10 to 18 million men between the ages of 40 to 70. Impotence affects about one out of every ten American men, and many of them don't seek help because they are embarrassed. Not only can it be embarrassing for the male, but for the female as well. Impotence may lead women to feel they are unattractive to their partner or that they cannot sexually satisfy their mates. A few years ago, most doctors thought that impotence was mainly psychological, but now it is believed that physical problems cause 50 to 80% of all erectile dysfunction.

We now known that a man's physical and psychological health, as well as his lifestyle, can all cause impotence. In order to achieve an erection, there are several parts of the body that must work together. An erection begins with both sensory and mental stimulation. The brain sends a message of sexual arousal through the nervous system to the nerves, which innervate the muscles of the penis. This message causes the muscles of the penis to relax, while the artery, which carries blood to the penis, expands to almost twice its size, increasing the blood flow into the penis.

The veins, which carry blood away from the penis, are blocked, causing blood to flow directly into the penis. This allows no blood to escape out of the penis, causing the penis to fill with blood and to become firm. If just one of these systems breaks down, it is very difficult to get or keep an erection. Sex is a very complicated process, involving many bodily systems. Sexual activity takes a lot of energy, and can drain the body of energy in a matter of seconds to minutes. In fact, sexual activity takes more energy from the body than any other physical activity.

Almost all men occasionally fail to get an erection at some time during their life, and this is considered normal, but when a man has trouble maintaining an erection about 25% of the time, he is considered impotent. Damage to arteries, veins, muscles, and nerves, often as the result of a disease, is the most common cause of impotence. Diseases such as diabetes, high blood pressure, kidney disease, MS, Parkinson's disease, alcoholism, atherosclerosis, and vascular disease make up more than 70% of the cases of impotence, which means that the majority of impotence is caused by what men eat.[68] It is estimated that physical factors account for about 80% of the cases of impotence.[69]

Surgery to remove certain cancers from the colon, rectum, urinary bladder, or prostate can cause impotence, because many of the nerves that control erections are damaged during these types of surgery. Many common medicines for high blood pressure, diabetes, depression, and ulcer drugs cause interference with blood flow and nerve impulses to the penis.[70]

Smoking and alcohol increase the risk for impotence. Excessive alcohol consumption can disrupt testosterone, male hormone, levels and lead to nerve damage.[71] Vascular disease such as hardening of the arteries (atherosclerosis) can affect blood flow to the penis, which makes it hard to achieve and sustain an erection.[72]

There are a variety of treatments for erectile dysfunction, including a vacuum device, which is used to create a vacuum of air that draws blood into the penis. Drugs can also be injected into the penis to increase blood flow. Rods and inflatable cylinders may also be implanted into the penis to achieve erections. Viagra is estimated to have helped about 70% of men with erectile dysfunction; they simply take Viagra one hour before sex, and it does the rest.

Man is the only species of animal that needs to take medicine to achieve an erection. Most causes of impotence are due to fat and cholesterol that has clogged up the artery leading to the penis.[73] As long as you eat fatty foods, the body will deposit fats in the arteries leading to the penis. The body has to put the excess fat somewhere, and puts it in all three of the arteries that supply blood to the organs needed for sex - arteries that supply the brain for sensation, the heart for blood, and the penis for ejaculation. When something goes wrong with just one of these systems, we have problems with impotence. For example, sometimes my mom would pour grease into the sink after cooking hamburgers or frying foods. After pouring grease and fat into the sink over a period of time, the grease would clog the pipes and water could not flow feely down the drain. The same happens to the artery innervating the penis after eating grease, fats, and cholesterol over a period time. It is similar to having a heart attack or a stroke, and in many cases, men would probably rather have a stroke or a heart attack, than be impotent.

There are many natural things a man can do to prevent impotence - exercise, limit or eliminate fat and cholesterol in his diet, stop drinking and smoking, and most importantly, eat low fat, high fiber foods. Men with erectile dysfunction are usually overweight and don't exercise. If you are suffering from impotence, do you eat lots of fried and fatty foods, excessive amounts of meats and dairy products, which are full of fats and cholesterol? Probably so. Do you drink lots of alcohol and smoke tobacco? Probably so. Do you have lots of stress, depression, and anxiety in your life? If so, the problem is not in your head, it is in your arteries and nerves, because of a deceitful diet. If you want to prevent impotence start to exercise on a regular basis, keep stress to a minimum, drink plenty of water, and eat a majority of God's Original Diet.

There are many other diseases that I did not discuss that occur due to The Standard American Diet. Most of them can all be avoided, if only we would change our diet and eat a majority of foods that God told us to eat. Notice there are many diseases, but they all come from the same sources. The same foods effect different people in different ways. Alcohol may cause impotence in one person, but may cause kidney disease in another. Excessive amounts of meats may cause a heart attack in one person, but may cause a stroke in another. Most diseases are the same; the only difference is that they occur in different parts of the body. All cancers, no matter where they occur, are the same and they can be prevented, whether they be skin, colorectal, breast, or prostate. Heart attacks, strokes, and impotence are all the same. They are all due to a buildup of fat in the arteries. Changing our diet and lifestyle can prevent colds, flu, and other mucus-forming illnesses.

The best way to prevent or treat these diseases is to eat the way God intended, stay active, reduce stress, and use all the spiritual aspects of health. When it comes to our health, it is time for us to stop putting our faith in man and start putting it in God. Only He knows what is good for His people, and He has already told us what is good for our health. It is up to us to follow his instructions, or pay the consequences with sickness and diseases.

> *Exodus 23:25 And ye shall serve the Lord your God and he shall bless thy bread, and thy water; and I will take sickness away from the midst of thee.*

VIII.
EATING THE WAY GOD INTENDED

People often ask me what I eat, and to give them a healthy meal plan. I eat very simple and my meals are pretty basic. I eat until I am full, and I do not stop eating until I have a satisfied and full feeling.

For breakfast I eat a variety of fruit. My breakfast consists of at least five of the following fruits:

Watermelons	Oranges
Apples	Pineapples
Mango	Banana
Kiwi	Green grapes
Red Grapes	Peaches
Tangerine	Dried Fruits
Prunes	Dates
Figs	Raisins

Apricot

For lunch I may snack on some raw nuts and seeds mixed with raisins. I eat a variety of the following raw nuts and seeds:

Peanuts	Cashews
Almonds	Pecans
Pignoli	Brazil Nuts
Flax seeds	Sunflower seeds

Sesame seeds

For lunch I may also have a vegetable salad, with some of the following vegetables:

Lettuce	Cucumbers
Celery	Tomato
Avocado	Green peppers
Raw Spinach	Broccoli
Cauliflower	Flax seeds
Onion	Sprouts
Carrots	Mushrooms

For dinner I eat at least four different vegetables from the list below with fresh legumes:

Broccoli	Peas
Cabbage	Fresh Corn
Butterbeans	All Green Leafy Vegetables
Squash	Baked Potato
Fresh lima beans	Fresh pinto beans
Asparagus	Cauliflower

Always try to eat fresh vegetables; the next best is frozen vegetables. Try not to eat vegetables and other foods in cans, because they have been preserved with salts, sugars, and other harmful chemicals.

Here is a list of foods that you can eat throughout the day. Alternate them daily because the earth provides a variety of foods that God has given man to eat.

FRUITS

Apples	Dates
Apricot	Figs
Avocado	Grapefruit
Blueberries	Lemon
Blackberry	Mango
Cranberry	Nectarine
Gooseberry	Oranges
Huckleberry	Papaya
Red and Black Raspberry	Peaches
Strawberry	Pears
Bananas	Persimmons
Cantaloupe	Pineapples
Red and Black Cherries	Plums
Currants	Prunes
Raisins	Tangerine
Lime	Watermelon
Olives	Rhubarb
Tomatoes	Pomegranate

VEGETABLES AND FRESH LEGUMES

Alfalfa	Asparagus
Green Beans	Beets
Broccoli	Green Peas
Brussel sprouts	Cabbage greens
Purple Hull Peas	Carrots
Cauliflower	Black eye Peas
Celery	Chives
Zucchini	Cucumbers
Dandelion	Mushrooms
Endive	Fennel
Collard Greens	Garlic
Horseradish	Artichokes
Kale	Leeks
Eggplant	Lettuce
Mustard greens	Lima Beans
Okra	Onions
Lentils	Parsley
Parsnips	Corn
Field Peas	Green and Red Peppers
Watercress	Potatoes
Sweet Potatoes	Butterbeans
Pumpkins	Radishes
Squash	Rutabagas
Spinach	Turnip Greens
Soybeans	Kidney Beans

Navy Beans

RAW NUTS and SEEDS

Almonds	Pecans
Cashews	Brazil
Walnuts	Pignolias (Aka pine nuts)
Hickory	Acorn
Chestnuts	Pistachio
Filberts	Macadamia
Raw Seeds	Sunflower
Pumpkin	Sesame
Flax	Squash

WHOLE GRAINS

Wheat	Oats
Barley	Corn
Millet	Rye
Rice	Buckwheat

BETTER FOOD SUBSTITUTES

Foods commonly used:	Better Substitutes:
White and brown sugars	Raw honey, dates, molasses, maple syrup
White bread	Wheat, rye, multigrain Ezekiel or any whole grain breads
Butter or margarine	Nut butters, avocado, Earth Balance and Spectrum natural butters (found at local health food stores)
Salt	Bragg Liquid Aminos
Cows milk	Mother's breast milk for infants and babies from birth to nine months. 8th Continent and Silk soy milk or rice milk
White rice	Brown rice
Chocolate	Carob (contains no caffeine)
Coffee	Water
White flour	Wheat flour, multigrain, oat grain, yellow or white corn meal (any unprocessed whole grain flour)
Vegetable oils, lard	Olive oil

BETTER FOOD SUBSTITUTES

Foods commonly used:	Better Substitutes:
White pasta	Whole wheat pasta, corn pasta (any whole grain pasta)
White crackers	Wheat crackers
French Fries	Baked potatoes
Fried potato chips	Baked potato chips, corn chips, chips that are salt free
Sugar coated cereals	Oatmeal, whole grain grits, brown rice, millett, whole grain cereals; if you have to put milk on cereals use soy, rice or almond milk
Bacon and sausage	Alternatives made from soy products
Meats	Alternatives made from soy products. (Be careful not to get genetically engineered foods commonly found in some Boca and Morning Star Products.)
Ice Cream	Ice cream made from soy or rice milk and ice cream made from real fruit. Soy Dream, Tofuti and Soy Delicious
Sodas, Coffee and Teas	Water and freshly squeezed fruit juice

BETTER FOOD SUBSTITUTES

Foods commonly used:	Better Substitutes:
Alcohol and wine	Freshly squeezed grape juice (no alcohol)
Sugary-flavored fruit drinks	Freshly squeezed fruit drinks
Cheeses and sour cream	Alternative cheeses made from soy, alternative sour cream made from tofu or soy. (Veggie Slice)
Peanut butter	Peanut, almond, and other nut butters that do not have hydrogenated fat added. There are many health food stores that let you grind nuts into butter. (Real peanut butter oils float above the butter.)
Ketchups	Use ketchups made from organic tomatoes with no salt or sugar.
Salad dressings	Use salad dressings that contain no vinegar, salt, sugar or other chemicals. (Nasoya Vegi-Dressing)
Vinegar	Organic apple cider vinegar
Jellies and jams	Use jelly and jams made with real fruit
Dried fruits preserved with sulfur	Eat dried fruits without preservatives

BETTER FOOD SUBSTITUTES

Foods commonly used:	Better Substitutes:
Fried chicken, turkey, and fish with scales and fins, e.g., salmon, grouper, tilapia, brim, bass, etc. They should be farm-raised without hormones and antibiotics	If you eat meat, eat baked meats no more than three times a week. (God gives us permission to eat these foods in Leviticus 11:9.)
Shrimp, lobster, catfish, oysters clams, crabs or non-scale fish	These foods should not be eaten. God calls them unclean in Leviticus 11:10-12, because they are scavengers and clean the waste in waters.

Remember, all of these alternative foods are not healthy, but they are better for the body than other man-made foods. The only foods that are healthy grow from the earth, and nothing should replace them. Honestly, if you do not grow food yourself you have no clue what you are getting. The government is allowing food to be genetically engineered without proper labeling, so the public doesn't know what they're eating. Many foods are labeled as natural, when they are not. If a food does not grow from the earth, it is not natural, meaning nature did not make it. Make common sense decisions when selecting your foods.

IX.
GOD'S ORIGINAL DIET ONE MONTH MEAL PLAN

Many people ask me to create a health plan for them, and are amazed at how simple it is. I include meats for meat-eaters, and I may include sweets if a person likes sweets. My meal plans include carbohydrates, proteins, sugar, and any other nutrients that so-called health experts tell you to stay away from. The only difference between the carbohydrates, proteins, and sugars that I recommend is that they come from God, and His foods will not harm you.

Here is my one-month plan for becoming healthier. It is very simple. If you follow this one-week plan for four weeks - one month - your health and energy will improve. Remember, the focus is not on weight loss, because when you start to eat healthier, weight loss will automatically follow. In some cases healthy eating may cause an increase in body weight, but if you follow this program, you are guaranteed to become healthier. Your energy will increase and your body weight will decrease. Don't stop eating this way when the month is over; make it a part of your everyday life. Become familiar with the foods that you are comfortable eating, and learn to listen to your body. Start adding exercise to your daily routine, especially walking, running, and sit-ups, to work out the heart. Only then will you begin giving your body the proper weapons - nutrients - to fight off sickness and disease.

Monday

Breakfast
√ Eat a variety of fresh raw fruits until you are full or satisfied. (Remember to eat watermelon first.) Fresh fruit is preferable to dried fruit. Choose from the list of fruits on page 131.
√ There should be no desire to drink.

Lunch
√ Eat a salad made with a variety of vegetables. If meat is desired on the salad, use chicken patties or nuggets made from soy products.
√ Use salad dressing with no vinegar, salt, or sugars.
√ If desired, snack on raw nuts.
√ If you want something to drink, remember, water is best.

Dinner

√ Eat at least three different types of vegetables, e.g., kale, mustard, collards, or other green leafy vegetables, broccoli and/or cauliflower, baked potato, peas, butterbeans, corn, or other vegetables. Choose from the list of vegetables on page 132.

√ Choose a starch such as a bake potato, a protein such as a bean and a green leaf such as turnips

√ Eat until full or satisfied.

√ Remember, no salt. If desired, use salt substitutes mentioned on page 134.

Exercise

√ Whenever you have free time during the day, go for a 20-minute walk or run, or do any other exercise you desire. The best time to exercise outdoors is in the morning or evening, when it is less humid and the sun's ray's are more comfortable.

<h2 style="text-align:center">Tuesday</h2>

Breakfast

√ Eat a variety of fresh raw fruits until you are full or satisfied. (Remember to eat watermelon first.) Fresh fruit is preferable to dried fruit. Choose from the list of fruits on page 131.

√ Another favorite of mine for breakfast is oatmeal with Earth Balance butter, raw pecans, and raisins.

Lunch

√ Eat a soy hamburger, with tomato, soy cheese, onions, and other ingredients you desire, along with a salad.

Dinner

√ Eat a variety of vegetables. Choose from the list of vegetables on page 132.

Wednesday

Breakfast
√   Eat a variety of fresh raw fruits, until you are full and satisfied, and whole grain grits with Earth Balance butter. (Remember to eat watermelon first.) Fresh fruit is preferable to dried fruit. Choose from the list of fruits on page 131.

Lunch
√   Eat a vegetable salad, meat alternative sandwich, and snack on raw nuts and seeds, e.g., cashews, pecans, flax, sunflower seeds, and almonds. Choose from the list of vegetables on page 132.

Dinner
√   Eat a mixed vegetable dinner, with broccoli, cauliflower, peppers, onions, squash, zucchini, olive oil, or other vegetables. Choose from the list of vegetables on page 132.

Exercise
√   Whenever you have free time during the day, go for a 20-minute walk or run, or do any other exercise you desire. The best time to exercise outdoors is in the morning or evening, when it is less humid and the sun's ray's are more comfortable.

Thursday

Breakfast
√   Eat 3 to 4 fresh raw fruits, then have some multigrain, buckwheat, oat grain, blu corn, or any other type of whole grain in the form of pancakes, waffles, or biscuits. If you love butter, use the butter alternative found at your local health food stores. Choose from a list of fruit listed on page 131.
√   Add bacon and sausage meat alternatives and you have a healthy traditional American breakfast.

Lunch
√   Eat raw nuts and/or vegetable salad.

Dinner

√ Eat vegetables, such as okra, cabbage, kale, corn, mashed potatoes, or other vegetables. Choose from the list of vegetables on page 132.

√ Eat alternative sweets or meats, if desired

Friday

Breakfast

√ Eat a variety of fresh raw fruits, and dried fruit if desired. Choose from the list of fruits on page 131.

Lunch

√ Drink freshly squeezed fruit juice made from oranges, apples, kiwi, grapes, grapefruit, and/or lemon, and you can even add vegetable juice from carrots, and celery.

Dinner

√ Eat a baked potato, with a variety of vegetables. Choose from the list of vegetables on page 132.

Exercise

√ Whenever you have free time during the day, go for a 20-minute walk or run, or do any other exercise you desire. The best time to exercise outdoors is in the morning or evening, when it is less humid and the sun's ray's are more comfortable.

Saturday

Breakfast

√ Eat your choice of freshly squeezed fruit juices or fresh raw fruit. Choose from the list of fruit on page 131.

Lunch

√ Eat a variety of raw nuts and seeds, along with a salad of fresh vegetables. Choose from a list of vegetables on page 132.

Dinner

√   Eat a variety of fresh vegetables, a soy hamburger, a baked potato or baked French fries, and salad. If desired, eat baked fish (optional). Choose from the list of vegetables on page 132.

Sunday

Breakfast

√   Eat your choice of freshly squeezed fruit juices, fresh fruit, or both. Choose from the list of fruit on page 131.

√   You can also have the traditional Sunday morning breakfast with sausage and bacon alternatives made from soy. Make pancakes, waffles, and biscuits from multigrain, buckwheat, blue corn, oat grain, or other whole-wheat flours.

Lunch

√   Snack on raw nuts and seeds, or have a vegetable salad, if desired. Choose from the list of vegetables on page 132.

Dinner

√   Eat a variety of traditional Sunday evening vegetables — mashed potatoes, cabbage, corn, or other vegetables with whole grain corn bread, and if you desire meat, have baked chicken (optional). Choose from the list of vegetables on page 132.

Remember, if you have to eat meat, limit meat to three times a week. Eating meat more than three times a week, in my opinion, is eating in excess. You should eat organic farm-raised chicken, turkey, and fish with scales, not because they are better, but because their meats are easier for the body to digest. Pigs and cows are very hard for the body to digest and eating them over a long period of time puts stress on the GI tract, not to mention the diseases they cause.

This is a one-week diet plan that you can use for the rest of your life. Try it for a month and see how it works for you. Remember, God's Original Diet never fails.

These foods are designed to make the body healthier and give the body more energy. If you desire, mix the foods up. If you desire to eat the traditional breakfast on a different day than the plan calls for, that's okay. And, if you desire to walk or run on Tuesday, Thursday, and Saturday, then go for it.

As long as you eat the way God intended and exercise at least two to three days a week, you will see improvement in your health. Use all the alternative foods as much as you desire. This is only an outline of the diet plan you should follow. You don't have to follow the meal plan exactly, but make sure that you eat fruits and vegetables every day of your life. Fruits and vegetables should make up at least 90% of your diet, which will give your body the proper nutrients it needs to fight off diseases.

X.
Conclusion

It is never God's will for any man to be sick. Man was never meant to suffer from cancer, diabetes, heart disease, stroke, and other diseases. In the beginning of time, man was supposed to live forever. He was to have a great life full of fun, sun, no worries, no disease, and no stress.

I hear many people saying that it must be God's will for them to have cancer, diabetes, arthritis, and other diseases. They say the Lord gave them the disease to increase their faith in Him, or that the Lord is putting them through a trial or test. The Lord very seldom gives His children diseases to see how much faith they have in Him. Would a mother give her son gasoline to drink when he is thirsty? Would a father give his daughter poison to eat? You might say, but that question does not make sense, because of course they would not. Well, saying that the Lord gave you a disease to test your faith in Him does not make sense either. Man brings most diseases upon himself.

When we do not abide by God's rules, we start to face troubles in our lives. We have been instructed to eat a majority of foods that grow from the earth, and when we start to eat a majority of foods that don't, we start developing sickness and disease. It is not God's fault that we do not follow his instructions; it is our own.

We must decrease the amount of deceitful food we eat if we want to prevent diseases and become healthy. I know how hard it is to stop eating red meats, and I know how hard it is to give up ice cream, cakes, and pies. I still taste sweets, such as cakes and pies, if my mom decides to bake. I even eat fish about once a month, but that's about as far as I go. Afterall, I am human and I have a desire to taste something sweet every once in a while, but I don't eat these foods on a daily basis. I have learned how to control my appetite and not let it control me.

The majority of your diet should consist of fruits, vegetables, raw nuts, seeds, and whole grains, and these are the least expensive foods that you can buy. You should drink mostly distilled water. If there is only one thing that you learn from reading this book, I want it to be that the majority of the foods you eat; 90% should be from God's Original Diet. Nothing in your diet should replace these foods. When you start to eat a majority of these foods, your health will be restored and your energy will improve.

Health comes from inside the body and shows on the outside. What you eat and put inside your body will eventually show on the outside. If you eat healthy foods that are full of life, your body will show energy and life on the outside. We have been taught by man that health comes from outside to inside the body. Man teaches us that we can take a vitamin or mineral pill, and it will restore our health on the inside. We have been taught that we can take medicine from the outside world, and it will make us healthier on the inside. This is far from the truth. We have been taking vitamins, supplements, and other medicine for years and they have not restored health. We have been following all kinds of diets for weight loss for years, and we have not lost weight in a healthy manner. We have been eating dead foods for years, and all we have to show for it are disease and death. So why not give God's Original Diet a try. What do you have to lose? God's Original Diet gives your body all the nutrients it needs, along with life and energy. It was here long before any diet and will be here long after all other diets.

When you eat the way God intended, you don't have to worry about diseases; you don't have to worry about cancer, you don't have to worry about diabetes. When you eat the way God intended, you don't have to worry about strokes, heart attacks, and impotence. If you are tired of being sick and diseased, if you are tired of being overweight, if you are tired of not having any energy, if you are just tired of being sick and tired, start eating foods that grow from the earth. It is not God's will for His children to be sick and diseased.

God came that we may have life and have life more abundantly. God is tired of seeing his children bound up with diseases that can be easily prevented. It is time for us to start living a healthy lifestyle and eating healthy foods. It is time for us to get off our behinds, and start walking, running, cycling, and exercising. It is time to restore our strength and take back our health.

Do not depend on man to give you health, for he has been trying to cure diseases for years, and has not cured one yet. Do not depend on man-made medicine, vitamins, minerals, and other so-called health pills. Sure, they have their place, but they never restore health. It is time that we depend on God for our health, for His diet has no side effects, and provides our body with great health, energy, life, and life more abundantly. If you are looking for health and looking for it in all the wrong places, give God's Original Diet a try.

Diseases that are linked to our diet are killing many people everyday, but God has given us a way to avoid sickness and disease. He has given us His diet to eat since the beginning of time. You may have been told by your doctor that your disease is genetic and that you inherited it from your parents and grandparents. You may have also been told that cancer, diabetes, high blood pressure, fibroids, or other diseases are in your future because your parents had them. Well, I have good news. Just because your grandparents, aunties, uncles, mother, or father has a disease or died from a disease, does not mean you will have or die from that disease. Everyone in your family eats the same unhealthy foods, don't exercise, and live the same unhealthy lifestyle, therefore, everyone in your family gets the same diseases. You now have the power to stop this generational curse of sickness in your family by obeying God's natural law, which instructs to eat the fruit of the tree and herbs of the field.

America is a very blessed nation, but we continue to suffer with health problems, and will continue to suffer until we start to eat the way God intended. Let's stop being a sick nation, let's start eating foods that grow from the earth. It is time for us to go back to God's Original Diet and only then will we see our health increase, and disease decrease.

In the beginning of time, man, Adam, was given a choice by God to eat foods from the garden, or to eat from the deceitful tree. Adam chose to eat the deceitful food, and death came upon him. Today, God is still giving us that choice, to eat from his Original Diet or to eat deceitful foods. Sadly, many are still choosing to eat the deceitful foods, and just like Adam, we all die before our time. Remember, the first sin involved food.

Today man has placed before you foods that give sickness, fatigue, disease, and death. God has placed before you foods that give health, strength, energy, and life. Now, you have a choice. Which foods will you eat? My prayer is that you choose life.

I pray this book has been a blessing to you. May God bless you with life, and may you have it more abundantly.

> *3 John:2 Beloved, I wish above all things that thou mayest prosper and be in health, even as thy soul prospereth.*

Notes

Chapter III: My People Are Destroyed For Lack of Knowledge

1.   H. Diamond and M. Diamond, Fit For Life II: Living Health (New York, New York: Warner Books, 1987), 67.

2.   Breastfeeding and the Use of Human Milk, American Academy of Pediatrics. (RE2729).

3.   H.B. Slade and S.A. Schwartz, "Mucosal Immunity: The Immunology of Breast Milk," Journal of Allergy and Clinical Immunology 80, no.3 (September 1987): 348-356.

4.   B. Ducan, "Exclusive Breastfeeding for at Least Four Months Protects Otitis Media," Pediatrics 91 (1993): 872-897.

5.   T.G. Merrett, "Infant Feeding and Allergy: Twelve Month Prospective Study of 500 Babies Born in Allergic Families," American Allergy (1988): 13- 20.

6.   E.G. White, Counsels on Diet and Foods (Takoma Park, Washington, DC: Review and Herald Publishing, 1938), 331.

7.   C. Marsden, "Cow's Milk May Raise Diabetes Risk in Some Children," Diabetes 49 (2000): 1657-1665.

8.   S.J. Kaplan, "Dietary Replacement in Preschool-aged Hyperactive Boys," Pediatrics 83 (1989): 7-17.

9.   G. Pamplona-Roger, M.D., Encyclopedia of Medicinal Plants (Colmenar Viejo, Madrid, Spain: Editorial Safeliz, 2001), 152.

10. E.G. White, Counsels on Diet and Foods (Takoma Park, Washington, D.C.: Review and Herald Publishing, 1938), 420-427.

11. Crack and Cocaine, National Institute on Drug Abuse (November 5, 1999).

12. A. Colman, "Possible Psychiatric Reactions to Monosodium Glutamate," New England Journal of Medicine 299 (1978): 26.

13. M.L. Sullivan, C.M. Martinez, P. Gennis, and E.J. Gallagher, "The Cardiac Toxicity of Anabolic Steroids," Progress in Cardiovascular Diseases 41(1) (1998): 1-15.

14. H. Silverman, Pharm.D., The Pill Book 8th Edition (New York, New York: Bantam Books, 1998), 1199-1201.

15. J. Parker, Crystal Meth & Other Stimulants: Maximum Speed, Do It Now

Foundation. Catalog no. 101 (October 2000).

16. E. Nadelmann, "Drug Prohibition in the United States: Costs, Consequences and Alternatives," Science (September 1, 1989) and C. Foster, CSM (September 18, 1989).
Mokdad, Ali H. PhD, Jones S. Marks, MD, MPH, Donna F. Stroup, PhD, "Actual Causes of Death in the United States 2000. Journal of the American Medical Association, March 10, 2004, Vol. 291, No. 10, P. 1242.

17. Dr. Julian Whitaker, "The Dangers of Overusing Pain Relievers," Health and Healing (May 1998).

18. T. Nordenberg, "Make No Mistake: Medical Errors Can be Deadly Serious," FDA Consumer Magazine (September-October 2000).

19. Regulating Pesticides in Food 78-80, National Research Council. Board on Agriculture. Table 3, 20-22.

20. F. Kuchler, "Regulating Food Safety: The Case of Animal Growth Hormones," National Food Review (July-December, 1989):26.

21. J. Robbins, "Diet for A New America" (Walpole, NH: Stillpoint Publishing, 1987), 48-72.

22. Ibid. 97-212.

23. J. Manson and P. Singer, Animal Factories (New York, New York: Harmony Books, 1990), 81-89.

24. C. Foreman and L. Carey, Public Comments on Food Safety and Inspection Service. U.S. Dept. of Agriculture, Food Safety and Inspection Service. Public Docket no. 83-008P, 53 Federal Register 48262 (November 30, 1988).

25. J. Rifkin, Beyond Beef: The Rise and Fall of the Cattle Culture, (New York, New York: Plume Book Publishing, 1992), 132-145.

26. Ibid. 132-145.

Chapter IV: Feed Me With Food Convenient For Me.

1. "FDA Announces Withdrawal of Fenfluramine and Dexfenfluramin (Fen-Phen)," New England Journal of Medicine 337(9) (August 28, 1997): 581-588.

2. John Robbins, The Food Revolution (Berkeley, CA: Conari Press, 2001), 66.

3. Ibid. 62-63.

4. J. McDougall, The McDougall Plan (Clinton, NJ: New Winn Publishing, 1983), 76-94.

5. H. Diamond and M. Diamond, Fit For Life II: Living Health (New York, New York: Warner Books, 1987), 234.

6. D. Ornish, Dr. Dean Ornish's Program for Reversing Heart Disease (New York, New York: Ballantine Books, 1996), 254-255.

7. J. McDougall, The McDougall Program For A Healthy Heart (New York, New York: Plume Publishing, 1998), 219-223.

8. J. Gainer, "Protein and Hardening of the Arteries," Science News (August 21, 1971).

9. Diamond op.cit. 234.

10. N.A. Breslau, L. Brinkley, K.D. Hill and Cy Pak, "Relationship of Animal Protein-rich Diet to Kidney Stone Formation," Journal Of Clinical Endocrinal Metabolism 66 (1988):140-146.

Chapter V: For They Are Deceitful Meat (Food)

1. Journal of the American Medical Association (January 26, 1994):280-283.

2. L. Massey Ph.D. and K.J. Wise, B.S., "The Effect of Dietary Caffeine on Urinary Excretion of Calcium, Magnesium, Sodium and Potassium in Healthy Young Females," Nutrition Research (January/February 1984):43.

3. J.E. James, "Caffeine and Health," Progress in Clinical Research 158 (Academic Press, 1991).

4. How to Help Your Patients Stop Using Tobacco: A National Cancer Institute Manual for the Oral Health Team, U.S. Department of Health and Human Services. National Institutes of Health Publication No. 963191 (1996).

5. C. King, M. Siegel, C. Celebucki and G. Connolly, "Adolescent Exposure to Cigarette Advertising in Magazines: An Evaluation of Brand-specific Advertising in Relation to Youth Readership," Journal of the American Medical Association 279, no. 7:520.

6. J.E. Henningfield, C. Cohen, and W.B. Pickworth, Psychopharmacology of Nicotine (1993).

7. "The Health Consequences of Smoking: Nicotine Addiction," A Report of the

Surgeon General. U.S. Department of Health and Human Services. Department of Health and Human Services Publication No. 96-3191 (1998).

8.   J.E. Harris, "Cigarette Smoke Components and Disease: Cigarette Smoke is More Than a Triad of Tar, Nicotine and Carbon Monoxide," National Cancer Institute Monographs 7:59-61.

9.   Reducing the Health Consequences of Smoking: 25 Years of Progress. A Report of the Surgeon General. U.S. Department of Health and Human Services. Department of Health and Human Services Publication No. (CDC) 89-8411 (1989).

10. J. Trop, Please Don't Smoke In Our House, (Chicago, IL: Natural Hygiene Press, 1976), 54-56.

11. Cigars: Health Effects and Trends, National Cancer Institute Communications Release. National Cancer Institute (April 10, 1998).

12. P.S. Blair, P.J. Fleming, D. Bensley, I. Smith, C. Bacon and E. Taylor, "Smoking and Sudden Infant Death Syndrome: Results from 1993-5 Case-control Study for Confidential Inquiry into Stillbirths and Deaths in Infancy," British Medical Journal 313:195-198.

13. Respiratory Health Effects of Passive Smoking: Fact Sheet, U.S. Environment Protection Agency (1993).

14. Mayo Clinic Healthy Information. http://www.mayoclinic.com/home?id=DS00184.

15. J. McDougal, The McDougall Program For A Healthy Heart (New York, New York: Plume Publishing, 1996), 115-118.

16. J. Robbins, Diet For A New America (Walpole, NH: Stillpoint Publishing 1987), 175.

17. H. Diamond and M. Diamond, Fit For Life II: Living Health (New York, New York: Warner Books, 1987), 234.

18. Breastfeeding and the Use of Human Milk, American Academy of Pediatrics (RE22729).

19. "Lactose and Cataracts in Humans: A Review," Journal of American Coll Nutrition 10, no. 1 (1991): 79-86.
20. "Geographic Variations of Senile Osteoporosis," Journal of Bone and Joint Surgery 52B (1970): 667.

21. Food, Nutrition, and the Prevention of Cancer: A Global Perspective. World

Cancer Research Fund/American Institute for Cancer Research. American Institute for Cancer Research (Washington D.C., 1997): 322.

22. L. Burby, "101 Reasons to Breastfeed your Child" ProMoM, Inc. http://www.promom.org/101/.

23. W.B. Grant, "Milk and Other Dietary Influences on Coronary Heart Disease," Alternative Medicine Review 3, no. 4: 281-294.

24. H.C. Gerstein, "Cow's Milk Exposure and Type 1 Diabetes Mellitus," Diabetes Care 17, no. 1 (January 1994):13-19.

25. Diamond op.cit. 331.

26. Robbins op.cit. 65.

27. McDougal op.cit. 34-51.

28. E. White, Counsels on Diet and Foods, (Takoma Park, Washington, DC: Review and Herald Publishing, 1938), 327-328.

29. R. Mendelsohn, MD. How to Raise a Healthy Child in Spite of Your Doctor, (New York, New York: Ballantine Books, 1984), 220-229.

30. J. McDougall, M.D., The McDougall Plan (Clinton, NJ: New Win Publishing, 1983), 114-116.

31. H. Shelton, "Health For The Millions," American Natural Hygiene Society (1968): 139-141.

32. "Protein and Salt: Calcium Thieves," Nutrition Health Review 35 (June 1985): 4.

33. A.J. Cohen and F.J.C. Roe, "Evaluation of the Aetiological Role of Dietary Salt Exposure in Gastric and Other Cancers in Humans," Food and Chemical Toxicology 35 (1997): 271-293.

34. Greeley, "A Pinch of Controversy Shakes Up Dietary Salt," Food And Drug Administration. http//www.fda.gov/fdac/features/1997/797_salt.html.

35. Dr. J. Gainer, "Protein and Hardening of the Arteries," Science News (August 21, 1971).

36. Cunningham, "Lymphomas and Animal Protein Consumption," Lancet 2 (November 27, 1976): 1184.

37. P. Hill, "Environmental Factors and Breast and Prostate Cancer," Cancer Research 41 (September 1981): 3817.

38. C. Fredericks, PhD., Arthritis: Don't Learn to Live with It (New York, New York: Grosset and Dunlap, 1981).

39. F. Coe, "Eating Too Much Meat Causes Major Cause of Renal Stones," Internal Medical News 12 (1979): 1.

Chapter VI: Who Satisfieth Thy Mouth With Good Things

1.   M. Morrow-Tlucak, R.H. Haude and C.B. Ernhart, "Breastfeeding and Cognitive Development in the First 2 Years of Life," Soc Science Medicine (1988): 635-639.

2.   A. Lucas, "Breast Milk and Subsequent Intelligence Quotient in Children Born Preterm," Lancet 339 (1992):261-262.

3.   R. Von Kries, "Breastfeeding and Obesity: Cross Sectional Study." BMJ 319 (July 17, 1999):147-150.

4.   Acta Paediatrica 85, no. 5 (May 1996):525-530.

5.   Zheng, "Lactation Reduces Breast Cancer Risk in Shandong Province, China" Am J of Epidemiology 152, no. 12:1129.

6.   S. Chua, S. Arulkumaran and I. Lim, "Influence of Breastfeeding and Nipple Stimulation on Postpartum Uterine Activity," Br J Obstet Gynaecol 101 (1994):804-805.

7.   R.D. Williams, "Breastfeeding Best for Babies," U.S. Food and Drug Administration Statement: http://www.fda.gov.

8.   A.K. Koutras, "Fecal Secretory Immunoglobulin A in Breast Milk vs. Formula Feeding in Early Infancy," Journal of Pediatric Gastro Nutrition (1989).

9.   Archives of Pediatric and Adolescent Medicine (July 1995).

10. Lactose Intolerance, National Institute of Health. Publication No. 98-2751 (April 1994).

11. Fruit Nutrition Information, Nutrition Facts for Fruit, http://www.thefruitpages.com.

12. "Vegetables and Fruits in Food," Nutrition and the Prevention of Cancer: A Global Perspective," World Cancer Research Fund and American Institute for Cancer Research, Chapter 63 (1997): 436-446.

13. Urology (2001) 58:47-52.

14. Journal of Nutrition 127 (1997):383-393.

15. G. Block, B. Patterson and A. Subar, "Fruit, Vegetables, and Cancer Prevention: A Review of the Epidemiological Evidence," Nutritional Cancer 18 (1992):1-9.

16. Diet Nutrition and Cancer, National Academy of Sciences (1982).

Chapter VII: The Spiritual Way to Health

1. A. Goldhamer, D.C., D. Lisle, PhD., S. Anderson, MD., and T. Campbell, PhD., "Medically Supervised Water-Only Fasting in the Treatment of Hypertension," Journal of Manipulative and Physiological Therapeutics 24, no. 5 (June 2001):335-339.

2. J. Fuhrman, MD., Fasting and Eating for Health, (Griffin, New York, New York: St. Martin's Press, 1995).

3. H. Shelton, Fasting Can Save Your Life, American Natural Hygiene Society, Inc. (1987).

4. R.E. Dustman, R. Emmerson, and D. Shearer, "Physical Activity, Age, and Cognitive-Neuropsychological Function," Journal of Aging and Physical Activity 2 (1994):143-181.

5. "Technical Review: Exercise and NIDDM," American Diabetes Association. Diabetes Care 13 (1990):785-789. *R.J. Barnard, T. Jung, and S.B. Inkeles, "Diet and Exercise in the Treatment of NIDDM: The Need for Early Emphasis," Diabetes Care 17 (1994):1469-1472.

6. C. Bouchard, J-P Despres, and A. Tremblay, "Exercise and Obesity," Obesity Research 1 (1993):133-147.*P. Bjorntorp, L. Sjostrom, and L. Sullivan, "The Role of Physical Exercise in the Management of Obesity."

7. L. Berstein, B.E. Henderson, R. Hanisch, J. Sullivan-Hallye and R.K. Ross, "Physical Exercise and Reduced Risk of Breast Cancer in Young Women," Journal of the National Cancer Institute 86 (1994):1403-1408.

8. W.H. Ettinger, Jr. and R.F. Afable, "Physical Disability from Knee Osteoarthritis: The Role of Exercise as an Intervention," Medicine and Science in Sports and Exercise, 26 (1994):1435-1440.

9. R.P. Donahue, R.D. Abbott, D.M. Reed, and K. Yano "Physical Activity and Coronary Heart Disease in Middle Aged and Elderly Men: The Honolulu Heart Program," American Journal of Public Health 78 (1988):683-685. *J.A. Berlin and G.A. Coldita, "A Meta-Analysis of Physical Activity in the Prevention of Coronary Heart Disease," American Journal of Epidemiology 132 (1990):612-628.

10. S.H. Allen, "Exercise Considerations for Postmenopausal Women with Osteoporosis," Arthritis Care and Research 7 (1994):205-214.

11. Dr. J. Maas, Power Sleep, (New York, New York: Harper Perennial, 1998), 3-17.

12. G.R. Elliott and C. Eisdorfer, Stress and Human Health (New York, New York; Springer Publishing, 1982).

13. J. F. Borsschot, G.R. Godaert, C.J. Heijnen, R.E. Ballieux, R.J. Benschop, M. Olff, and M. De Smet, "Influence of Life Stress on Immunological Reactivity to Mild Psychological Stress," Psychosomatic Medicine 56 (1994):216-224.

14. "Drinking Water Contaminants," EPA Office of Water, http://www.epa.gov/safewater/hfacts.html.

15. J. Rifkin, Beyond Beef; The Rise and Fall of the Cattle Culture (New York, New York: Plumb Publishing, 1993),1,186,221.

16. K. Cantor, "Drinking Water Source and Chlorination Byproducts in Iowa. 111. Risk of Brain Cancer," American Journal of Epidemiology 150 (1999):552-560.

17. "Quantification of Cancer Risk from Exposure to Chlorinated Water," U.S. EPA. Office of Science and Technology. Office of Water (1998).

18. R.D. Morris, "Chlorination, Chlorination By-products, and Caner: A Meta-analysis," American Journal of Public Health 82 (1992):955-963.

19. "Drinking Water Contaminants," http://www.epa.gov/safewater/hfacts.html.

20. Rifkin op.cit. 218-219.

21. L.A.G. Ries, "Seer Cancer Statistics Review 1973-1977," National Cancer Institute.

22. L. Gross, "The Hidden Life of Bottled Water," Sierra Magazine (May 1999).

23. "Drinking Water Contaminants," http://www.epa.gov/safewater/hfacts.html.

24. "Ozone Layer," http://www.encyclopedia.com/articles/09732.

25. "Lack of Light Causes High Blood Pressure," Hypertension 30 (1997):150-156.

26. "The Sunlight on your Body," Principles of Health, http://www.pathlights.com/nr_encyclopedia/00prin4b.htm.

27. "Sunlight Exposure Beneficial In Multiple Sclerosis," Occupational Environmental Medicine 57 (2000):418-421.

28. R. Holden, Laughter, The Best Medicine (Hammersmith, London: Thorsons, 1993), 33-42.

29. "How Anger Affects Your Health," University of California Berkeley Wellness Letter 8 (January 1992).

Chapter VIII: For I am the Lord that Healeth Thee

1.   A. Ludington, M.D. and H. Diehl, Health Power: Health by Choice Not Chance (Hagerstown, MD: Review and Herald Publishing, 2000),64-65.

2.   A. Hartz, "Smoking, Coronary Artery Occlusion," Journal of the American Medical Association 246 (1981):851.

3.   W. Kempner, "Compensation of Renal Metabolic Dysfunction," North Carolina Medical Journal 8 (1947):128.

4.   A. Ludington, M.D. and H. Diehl, Health Power (Hagerstown, MD:Review and Herald Publishing, 2000), 45

5.   J. McDougall, M.D., The McDougall Program for a Healthy Heart (New York, New York: Plumb Publishing, 1998), 49.

6.   K. Zane, M.D., Sunlight Could Save Your Life (Penryn, California: World Health Publications, 1980),51-53.

7.   J. Hoover, N.D., Natural Medicine (Anaheim, CA: KNI Printer Inc., 1993), 31-32.

8.   D. Jablons et al., "Neoplasms of the Lung", In LW Way, G.M. Doherty, eds Current Surgical Diagnosis and Treatments, 11th ed (2003):395-407.

9.   H. Diamond and M. Diamond, Fit for Life II: Living Health (New York, New York: Warner Books, 1987), 76-78.

10. M.S. Chestnutt and T.J. Predergast, Pulmonare Neoplasms: Current Medical Diagnosis and Treatment, 42nd ed. (New York, New York: McGraw Hill, 2003), 2265-272.

11. W.J. Gradishsar, Diseases of the Breast, 2nd ed. (Philadelphia: Lippincott Williams and Wilkins, 2000), 661-667.

12. L. Bernstein and B.E. Henderson, "Physical Exercise and Reduced Risk of Breast Cancer in Young Women," Journal of the National Cancer Institute 86 (1994):

1403-1408.

13. S. A. Smith-Warner, "Alcohol and Breast Cancer in Women," Journal of the American Medical Association 279, no. 7 (1998): 535-539.

14. J.B. Barnett, "The Relationship between Obesity and Breast Cancer Risk," Nutrition Reviews 61, no. 2 (2003): 73-75.

15. M.D. Holmes, "Association of Dietary Intake of Fat and Fatty Acids with Risk of Breast Cancer," Journal of the American Medical Association 281, no. 10 (1999): 914-919.

16. E. Stefani, Meat Intake, "Heterocyclic Amines and Risk of Breast Cancer: A Case Control Study in Uruguay," Cancer Epidemio, Biomarkers, Prev. 6 (1997): 573-581.

17. G. Pamplona-Rodger, M.D., Encyclopedia of Foods and Their Healing Power Vol. 2, (Colmenar Viejo, Madrid, Spain: Editorial Safeliz, 2001), 264-274.

18. Ibid. 275-277.

19. Zheng et al., "Lactation Reduces Breast Cancer Risk in Shandong Province, China," American Journal of Epidemiology 152, no. 12: 1129.

20. N. Breslow, C.W. Chan and G. Dhom, "Latent Carcinoma of Prostate at Autopsy in Seven Areas," International Journal of Cancer 20(1977):680-8.

21. B. Armstrong and R. Doll, "Environmental Factors and Cancer Incidence and Mortality in Different Countries, with Special Reference to Dietary Practices," International Journal of Cancer 15 (1975):617-31.

22. F.L. Apperly, "The Relation of Solar Radiation to Cancer Mortality in North America," Cancer Research 1 (1941):191.

23. H. Seidel, J. Ball, and J. Dain, Mosby's Guide to Physical Exam, 3rd ed. (St. Louis, MO: Mosby, 1995), 524.

24. Ibid. 524.

25. Pamplona-Rodger op.cit. 374-377.

26. E. Bien, "The Relation of Dietary Nitrogen Consumption to the Rate of Uric Acid Synthesis in Normal and Gouty Men," Journal Clin Invest 32 (1953): 778.

27. Pamplona-Rodger op.cit. 317-318.

28. N. Zollner, "Diet and Gout," Proceedings of 9th Int Congr Nutr Mexico 1 (1972):267.

29. "Dr. Spock Sours on Cow Milk for Babies," Toronto Star (September 30, 1992).

30. J. Barnard, "Response of Non-Insulin Dependant Diabetic Patients to an Intensive Program of Diet and Exercise," Diabetes Care 5 (July/August 1982):370.
31. Lundington op.cit. 57.

32. G. Lewinnek, M.D., "The Significance and a Comparative Analysis of the Epidemiology of Hip Fractures," Clinical Orthopedics and Related Research 152 (October 1980):35.

33. E. Blume, "Protein," Nutrition Action 14 (March 1987):1.

34. R. Heaney, "Effects of Nitrogen, Phosphorus and Caffeine on Calcium Balance in Women," Journal of Laboratory and Clinical Medicine 99 (1982):46.

35. D. Feskanich, W.C. Williet, M.J. Stampfer, and G.A. Colditz, "Milk, Dietary Calcium and Bone Fractures in Women: A 12 year Prospective Study," American Journal of Public Health 87 (1997):992-7.
a.   *R.G. Cumming and R.J. Klineberg, "Case Control Study of Risk Factors for Hip Fractures in the Elderly," American Journal of Epidemiology 139 (1994):493-505.

36. H. Daniell, M. D., "Osteoporosis of the Slender Smoker: Vertebral Compression Fractures and Loss of Metacarpal Cortex in Relation to Post Menopausal Cigarette Smoking and Lack of Obesity," Archives of Internal Medicine 136 (March 1976):298.

37. "Smoking, Alcohol and Bone Degeneration," Nutrition Health Review 5 (June 1985):4.

38. S. Eastman, "Medications and Bone Loss," Nutrition Health Review 35 (June 1985):5.

39. Diamond op.cit. 55.

40. J. Aloia, "Prevention of Involution Bone Loss by Exercise," Annals of Internal Medicine 9 (1978): 356.

41. Z. Kime, M.D. Sunlight, (Penryn, California: World Health Publications, 1981).

42. D. Day Baird, "Highly Cumulative Incidence of Uterine Leiomyoma in Black and White Women: Ultrasound Evidence," American Journal of Obstetrics and Gynecology 188, no. 1 (2003): 100-107.

43. Ibid. 100-107.

44. Ibid. 100-107.

45. S. Lark, M.D., Fibroids Tumors and Endometriosis Self Help Book, (Berkley, CA: Celestial Arts, 1995).

46. McDougall op.cit. 246.

47. "What You Can Do to Prevent or Manage Fibroids," Essence Magazine (September 1, 2003):96.

48. W. Richardson, M.D. and J. Richardson, MBA, "Uterine Fibroids: The Epidemic," Atlanta Clinic of Preventive Medicine, Inc.) www.acpm.net

49. Ibid. 4.

50. Diamond op.cit. 1.

51. S. L. Bahna, M.D., Allergies to Milk, (New York, New York: Grune & Stratton, 1980). *P.D. Buisseret, "Common Manifestations of Cow's Milk Allergy in Children," Lancet 1 (February 11, 1978):304. *J. Tommori and H. Lehotzky, "Study of the Frequency of Cow's Milk Sensitivity in the Families of Milk-Allergic and Asthmatic Children," Acta Allergol 28 (July 1973):107.

52. A. Urisu, "Allergenic Activity of Heated and Ovomucoid Depleted Egg White," Journal Allergy of Clinical Immunology 100 (1997): 171-176.
a.   *A. Norgaard, "Egg and Milk Allergy in Adults: Diagnosis and Characterization," Allergy 47 (1992):503-509.
b.   *A. Moreno-Ancillo and M.T. Caballero, "Allergic Reactions to Anisakis Simplex Parasitizing Seafood," Annal Allergy Asthma Immunology 79 (1997): 246-250.

53. A.K. Koutras, "Fecal Secretory Immunoglobulin A in Breast Milk vs. Formula Feeding in Early Infancy," Journal of Pediatric Gastro Nutrition (1989).

54. Hoover op.cit. 84.

55. Ibid. 221.

56. Ibid. 240.

57. P. O'Conor, "Key Issues in the Diagnosis and Treatment of Multiple Sclerosis: An overview," Neurology 59, no. 6, Supplement 3 (2002).

58. B. Agranoff, "Diet and the Geographical Distribution of Multiple Sclerosis," Lancet 2 (November 2, 1974):1061.

59. F. Oski, M.D., Don't Drink Your Milk, (Syracruse: Mollica Press, LTD., 1983), 73-75.

60. J. Chen, et al., "The Metabolic Syndrome and Chronic Kidney Disease in U.S. Adults," Annals of Internal Medicine 140, no. 3 (2004):167-175.

61. D. Foque et al., "Low-Protein Diets for Chronic Renal Failure in Non Diabetic Adults," Cochrane Database of Systematic Reviews 1, Oxford: Update Software.

62. F. Derrick, "Kidney Stone Disease: Evaluation and Medical Management," Postgraduate Medicine 66 (1979):115. *F. Derrick, Jr. M.D. and W. Carter III, M.D., "Kidney Stone Disease: Evaluation and Medical Management," Postgraduate Medicine 66 (October 1979): 115.

63. H. Sarles, "Diet and Cholesterol Gallstones," Digestion 17 (1978):121.

64. A. Walker, "Dental Caries and Sugar Intake," Lancet 2 (1975):765.*R. Harris, "Biology of the Children of Hopewood House, Bowral, Australia: Observations on Dental Caries Experience Extending Over Five Years," (1957-61).

65. V.T. Martin and M.M. Behbehani, "Toward a Rational Understanding of Migraine Trigger Factors," Medical Clinics of North America 85, no. 4 (2001): 911-941.

66. Ibid. 911-941.

67. Ibid. 911-941.

68. C.A. Derby et al., "Modifiable Risk Factors and Erectile Dysfunction: Can Lifestyle Changes Modify Risk?" Urology 56, no. 2 (2000): 302-306.

69. R. Webber, "Erectile Dysfunction," Clinical Evidence 10 (2003): 1003-1011.

70. The Pill Book, 8th ed., 6,78,106,115,161,217

71. What Increases Your Risk for Erectile Dysfunction (Boise, ID: Healthwise Incorporated, 2006).

72. McDougall op.cit. 50.

73. H. Lyman, "Mad Cowboy, The Plain Truth from the Cattle Rancher Who Won't Eat Meat," (New York, New York: Scribner, 1998), 36.

God's Original Diet

Index

glucose 30, 35, 44, 104, 105, 106, 107

God 1, 2, 3, 4, 5, 6, 8, 13, 14, 19, 20, 21, 22, 25, 26, 35, 39, 41, 42, 47, 51, 52, 54, 55, 56, 57, 59, 70, 77, 78, 81, 83, 95, 97, 98, 99, 103, 104, 119, 123, 126, 129, 130, 131, 133, 135, 137, 138, 139, 141, 143, 145, 146

grains 5, 19, 25, 32, 52, 64, 84, 86, 97, 98, 121, 133, 144

grapes 45, 31, 130, 141

grits 9, 135, 140

H

halitosis 75

hamburger 4, 17, 19, 40, 139, 142

headache 2, 10, 12, 26, 54, 118, 125, 126

heart attack 4, 5, 23, 40, 63, 83, 84, 89, 90, 106, 129

heartburn 83, 91, 92

herbs 6, 14, 47, 146

heroin 28

high blood pressure 2, 4, 14, 20, 23, 36, 37, 40, 57, 58, 79, 81, 84, 85, 86, 87, 88, 106, 121, 122, 126, 128, 145, 154

hormones 8, 15, 32, 33, 42, 80, 89, 97, 126, 137, 148

hospital 7, 18, 19

hypertension 49, 81, 84, 85, 86, 153, 154

hysterectomy 109, 113

I

illegal 10, 11, 12, 14, 26, 27, 28, 93

immune system 8, 32, 42, 60, 73, 74, 114, 115, 116, 117, 118

impotence 29, 58, 97, 106, 127, 128, 129, 145

infertility 29, 112

insecticides 65, 68

iron 15, 33, 44, 46, 48, 49, 50, 51, 52, 113

J

joints 36, 45, 64, 68, 100, 101, 102

K

kidney failure 103, 121, 122

kidney stones 40, 123, 124

kidneys 19, 23, 26, 27, 29, 45, 46, 49, 56, 57, 64, 68, 71, 85, 86, 105, 112, 121, 122, 123

Kool-aid 4, 31, 59, 69, 70, 92, 102, 119, 124, 125

L

laughter 74, 155

leeks 49, 132

legal 10, 11, 12, 14, 26, 27, 28, 30, 85, 93

legumes 5, 24, 52, 53, 121, 131, 132

lemons 45

lentils 52, 132

lettuce 48, 49, 130, 132

limes 45

liver 10, 13, 17, 30, 45, 48, 49, 56, 57, 58, 68, 76, 79, 89, 106, 108, 123

love 1, 21, 22, 55, 72, 73, 88, 122, 140

lunch 4, 14, 17, 18, 37, 40, 130, 138, 139, 140, 141, 142

lung cancer 30, 65, 92, 93, 94, 96

M

magnesium 44, 46, 48, 49, 50, 51, 52, 110, 121, 149

male hormones 97

marijuana 10, 28

massage 64, 74

meal plans 138

melons 44

migraines 116, 125, 126

milk 80, 82, 105, 111, 115, 118, 119, 120, 121, 124, 126, 134, 135, 147, 150, 151, 152, 157, 158

millet 9, 52, 133

minerals 6, 8, 13, 17, 34, 35, 37, 40, 42, 44, 45, 46, 47, 48, 49, 51, 52, 67, 84, 93, 110, 111, 121, 145

Multiple Sclerosis 33, 72, 119, 154, 158

muscles 3, 8, 9, 48, 60, 61, 62, 63, 64, 68, 71, 76, 84, 86, 89, 102, 104, 110, 112, 114, 123, 125, 126, 127, 128

stress 12, 14, 19, 26, 41, 58, 62, 63, 64, 67, 68, 71, 73, 74, 76, 82, 83, 84, 86, 87, 88, 91, 94, 101, 102, 103, 108, 112, 113, 114, 118, 119, 121, 123, 125, 126, 127, 129, 142, 144, 154
stroke 4, 5, 15, 18, 23, 29, 37, 40, 63, 82, 87, 88, 89, 106, 129, 144
sugar 99, 103, 104, 105, 106, 107, 108, 125, 135, 136, 138, 159
sugar cane 46

T

tea 4, 18, 64, 84, 88, 111, 112, 114
teeth 8, 29, 31, 48, 49, 50, 67, 68, 110, 115, 116, 124, 125
thyroid 79
tobacco 11, 27, 28, 82, 91, 93, 94, 129, 149
tomato 130, 139
toxins 26, 43, 47, 56, 57, 58, 60, 61, 62, 63, 65, 66, 68, 71, 73, 74, 75, 76, 80, 86, 113
trans fat 33, 90
tuberculosis 58
tumors 13, 19, 37, 49, 58, 75, 79, 94, 95, 96, 112, 113, 126, 157

U

ulcers 13, 29, 49, 56, 63, 91
unsaturated fat 46, 50, 51, 90
urination 65, 68, 96, 105, 106, 122
uterus 42, 112, 113

V

vagina 96
vascular disease 128
vegetables 1, 2, 3, 4, 5, 6, 9, 17, 19, 24, 25, 34, 35, 36, 37, 40, 46, 47, 82, 84, 86, 90, 91, 92, 95, 96, 97, 98, 108, 111, 112, 113, 114, 121, 123, 125, 127, 130, 131, 132, 138, 139, 140, 141, 142, 143, 144, 152, 153
vegetarian 6, 40
viruses 8, 63, 73, 74, 80, 100, 105, 116 117, 118
vitamin A 13, 47, 48
vitamin D 30, 72, 89, 90, 97, 112
vitamins 3, 6, 8, 13, 14, 17, 23, 34, 35, 37, 40, 42, 44, 45, 46, 47, 48, 49, 50, 51, 52, 60, 84, 95, 97, 121, 145
vomiting 56, 76, 83, 98, 122, 123, 125, 126

W

walking 23, 30, 60, 61, 64, 66, 86, 87, 88, 90, 91, 96, 100, 102, 107, 111, 113, 116, 120, 138, 145
walnuts 50, 133
water 4, 15, 16, 23, 26, 31, 32, 33, 35, 36, 40, 44, 45, 46, 47, 48, 49, 52, 53, 54, 55, 57, 67, 68, 69, 70, 92, 98, 99, 103, 128, 129, 134, 135, 138, 144, 153, 154
water pollution 68
whole grains 5, 19, 25, 52, 64, 86, 98, 121, 133, 144
whole wheat 135